Essential MCQs
on clinical pharmacology
and therapeutics

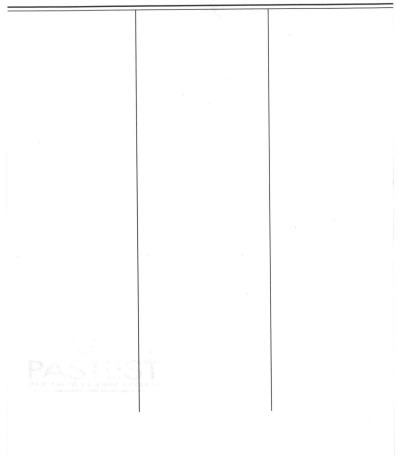

This book is due for return on or before the last date shown below.

Essential MCQs
on clinical pharmacology
and therapeutics

Delilah Hassanally BSc MBBS MSc FRCS
Specialist Registrar Surgery
North East Thames Rotation

Balvinder Singh Wasan BSc MBBS MRCP
Specialist Registrar Cardiology
St Mary's Hospital
London

With special thanks to
Rema Kaur Wasan BA MBBS MA MRCP FRCR
Consultant Radiologist
King's College Hospital
London

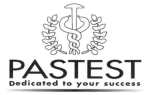

PASTEST
Dedicated to your success

© 2003 PASTEST Ltd
Egerton Court
Parkgate Estate
Knutsford
Cheshire
WA16 8DX
Telephone: 01565 752000

First published 2003

ISBN 1 901198 32 4

A catalogue record for this book is available from the British Library.

The information contained within this book was obtained by the author from
reliable sources. However, while every effort has been made to ensure its
accuracy, no responsibility for loss, damage or injury occasioned to any person
acting or refraining from action as a result of information contained herein can be
accepted by the publishers or author.

PasTest Revision Books and Intensive Courses

PasTest has been established in the field of postgraduate medical education since
1972, providing revision books and intensive study courses for doctors preparing
for their professional examinations. Books and courses are available for the
following specialties:

**MRCGP, MRCP Part 1 and 2, MRCPCH Part 1 and 2, MRCPsych, MRCS, MRCOG,
DRCOG, DCH, FRCA, PLAB.**

For further details contact:

PasTest, Freepost, Knutsford, Cheshire WA16 7BR
Tel: 01565 752000 Fax: 01565 650264
www.pastest.co.uk   enquiries@pastest.co.uk

Typeset by Vision Typesetting, Manchester
Printed by MPG Books Limited, Bodmin, Cornwall

Contents

Introduction

There are many multiple choice question books for postgraduate examinations. For years undergraduates have been forced to struggle with these as there is very little available for their needs.

Our aim is to provide real style practice examination questions at the appropriate level for undergraduates sitting pharmacology examinations.

This book consists of three test papers, answers and detailed teaching notes. The questions are as 'real' as can be; they include questions that have been remembered by students as they came out of their examination.

There is a natural tendency to recall the harder and more confusing questions, but rather than discarding these or simplifying them, we have deliberately included these and so the pass mark for each paper is probably a little less than 50%. We hope medical students will use this to their advantage; everyone will get the easy questions right, but the student who enters the examination having done the more difficult questions should not just pass, but pass well.

Delilah Hassanally
Balvinder Wasan

MCQ
Examination Technique

Before sitting an MCQ examination, you will need to know how many questions are likely to be on the paper and how long you will be given to complete it. So you will be able to assess the approximate amount of time that can be spent on each question. Pacing yourself accurately during the examination to finish on time, or with time to spare, is essential.

In MCQ examinations you must read the question (both stem and items A–E) carefully. Take care not to mark the wrong boxes and think very carefully before making a mark on the answer sheet. Regard each item as being independent of every other item – each refers to a specific quantum of knowledge. The item (or the stem and the item taken together) make up a statement. You are required to indicate whether you regard this statement as 'True' or 'False'. Look only at a single statement when answering – disregard all the other statements presented in the question. They have nothing to do with the item you are concentrating on.

As you go through the questions, you can either mark your answers immediately on the answer sheet or you can mark them on the question paper and then transfer them to the answer sheet. If you adopt the second approach you must take great care not to make any errors and not to run out of time, since you will not be allowed extra time to transfer marks to the answer sheet. The answer sheet must always be marked neatly and carefully according to the instructions given. Careless marking is probably one of the commonest causes of rejection of answer sheets by the document reader.

- Do as many good quality practice papers as possible. This will help you to identify your strengths and weaknesses in time for further study. You can also use the Revision Index at the back of this book to find questions on specific areas, so that after you have done some reading you can test your knowledge.
- With the three exams provided in this book be strict with yourself and work under realistic exam conditions. You should develop an understanding of your own work rate so that you know how much time you can spend on each question.
- Read each question several times. Nobody at this vital stage in their career should be wasting marks because they misread or misunderstood the question.
- Each exam in this book contains 50 questions.
- If you have to guess the answer to a question, put a special mark next to it. You will then be able to find out if you are a good guesser. This is especially important if your examination is negatively marked, i.e. marks will be deducted for incorrect answers. It is important to *know* what you know as well as what you don't know.

Sample Answer Sheet

UNIVERSITY OF LONDON Management Systems Division

MULTIPLE-CHOICE EXAMINATION ANSWER SHEET

Candidate No.	Test No.	College No.

DATE.........

SURNAME.........

FIRST NAME(S).........

Instructions: Use the HB pencil provided. To make an answer draw a single horizontal line along the dotted line above the appropriate letter or number. To answer 'TRUE' draw your line above the capital letter in the upper row. To answer 'FALSE' draw your line above the lower case letter in the lower row. For example:

[A] for 'TRUE'   [A] for 'FALSE'
[a]   [a]

If you change your mind and wish to cancel a completed answer, draw another line below the letter or number, along the dotted line. Do not rub out.

Candidate No. / Test No. / College No. number grids:

|0| |0| |0| |0| |0| |0| |0| |0| |0| |0|
|1| |1| |1| |1| |1| |1| |1| |1| |1| |1|
|2| |2| |2| |2| |P| |2| |2| |2| |2| |2|
|3| |3| |3| |3| |3| |3| |3| |3| |3|
|4| |4| |4| |4| |4| |4| |4| |4| |4|
|5| |5| |5| |5| |5| |5| |5| |5| |5|
|6| |6| |6| |6| |6| |6| |6| |6| |6|
|7| |7| |7| |7| |7| |7| |7| |7| |7|
|8| |8| |8| |8| |8| |8| |8| |8| |8|
|9| |9| |9| |9| |9| |9| |9| |9| |9|

Shown below is the correct method of completion, the correct method of cancellation/alteration and examples of various incorrect methods of completion.

CORRECT METHOD OF COMPLETION

[A] [A]
True =   False =
[a] [a]

CORRECT METHOD OF CANCELLATION/ALTERATION

To cancel a response, draw a line below the letter. Do not rub out. Thus:

[A] or [A] = Cancelled
[a]   [a]

To alter a response, first cancel. Then draw a line above the other letter. Thus:

[A] [A]
False =   True =
[a] [a]

INCORRECT METHODS OF COMPLETION

Too faint   [A]
Slanted   [A]
Too low   [A]
Too high   [A]
Into next box [A][B]
Too short   [A] [A] [A]
Isolated cancellation [A]
DETERMINATE TYPE T

Answer grid (questions 1–60):

1 [A] [B] [C] [D] [E] / [a] [b] [c] [d] [e]
2 [A] [B] [C] [D] [E] / [a] [b] [c] [d] [e]
3 [A] [B] [C] [D] [E] / [a] [b] [c] [d] [e]
4 [A] [B] [C] [D] [E] / [a] [b] [c] [d] [e]
5 [A] [B] [C] [D] [E] / [a] [b] [c] [d] [e]
6 [A] [B] [C] [D] [E] / [a] [b] [c] [d] [e]
7 [A] [B] [C] [D] [E] / [a] [b] [c] [d] [e]
8 [A] [B] [C] [D] [E] / [a] [b] [c] [d] [e]
9 [A] [B] [C] [D] [E] / [a] [b] [c] [d] [e]
10 [A] [B] [C] [D] [E] / [a] [b] [c] [d] [e]
11 [A] [B] [C] [D] [E] / [a] [b] [c] [d] [e]
12 [A] [B] [C] [D] [E] / [a] [b] [c] [d] [e]
13 [A] [B] [C] [D] [E] / [a] [b] [c] [d] [e]
14 [A] [B] [C] [D] [E] / [a] [b] [c] [d] [e]
15 [A] [B] [C] [D] [E] / [a] [b] [c] [d] [e]
16 [A] [B] [C] [D] [E] / [a] [b] [c] [d] [e]
17 [A] [B] [C] [D] [E] / [a] [b] [c] [d] [e]
18 [A] [B] [C] [D] [E] / [a] [b] [c] [d] [e]
19 [A] [B] [C] [D] [E] / [a] [b] [c] [d] [e]
20 [A] [B] [C] [D] [E] / [a] [b] [c] [d] [e]
21 [A] [B] [C] [D] [E] / [a] [b] [c] [d] [e]
22 [A] [B] [C] [D] [E] / [a] [b] [c] [d] [e]
23 [A] [B] [C] [D] [E] / [a] [b] [c] [d] [e]
24 [A] [B] [C] [D] [E] / [a] [b] [c] [d] [e]
25 [A] [B] [C] [D] [E] / [a] [b] [c] [d] [e]
26 [A] [B] [C] [D] [E] / [a] [b] [c] [d] [e]
27 [A] [B] [C] [D] [E] / [a] [b] [c] [d] [e]
28 [A] [B] [C] [D] [E] / [a] [b] [c] [d] [e]
29 [A] [B] [C] [D] [E] / [a] [b] [c] [d] [e]
30 [A] [B] [C] [D] [E] / [a] [b] [c] [d] [e]
31 [A] [B] [C] [D] [E] / [a] [b] [c] [d] [e]
32 [A] [B] [C] [D] [E] / [a] [b] [c] [d] [e]
33 [A] [B] [C] [D] [E] / [a] [b] [c] [d] [e]
34 [A] [B] [C] [D] [E] / [a] [b] [c] [d] [e]
35 [A] [B] [C] [D] [E] / [a] [b] [c] [d] [e]
36 [A] [B] [C] [D] [E] / [a] [b] [c] [d] [e]
37 [A] [B] [C] [D] [E] / [a] [b] [c] [d] [e]
38 [A] [B] [C] [D] [E] / [a] [b] [c] [d] [e]
39 [A] [B] [C] [D] [E] / [a] [b] [c] [d] [e]
40 [A] [B] [C] [D] [E] / [a] [b] [c] [d] [e]
41 [A] [B] [C] [D] [E] / [a] [b] [c] [d] [e]
42 [A] [B] [C] [D] [E] / [a] [b] [c] [d] [e]
43 [A] [B] [C] [D] [E] / [a] [b] [c] [d] [e]
44 [A] [B] [C] [D] [E] / [a] [b] [c] [d] [e]
45 [A] [B] [C] [D] [E] / [a] [b] [c] [d] [e]
46 [A] [B] [C] [D] [E] / [a] [b] [c] [d] [e]
47 [A] [B] [C] [D] [E] / [a] [b] [c] [d] [e]
48 [A] [B] [C] [D] [E] / [a] [b] [c] [d] [e]
49 [A] [B] [C] [D] [E] / [a] [b] [c] [d] [e]
50 [A] [B] [C] [D] [E] / [a] [b] [c] [d] [e]
51 [A] [B] [C] [D] [E] / [a] [b] [c] [d] [e]
52 [A] [B] [C] [D] [E] / [a] [b] [c] [d] [e]
53 [A] [B] [C] [D] [E] / [a] [b] [c] [d] [e]
54 [A] [B] [C] [D] [E] / [a] [b] [c] [d] [e]
55 [A] [B] [C] [D] [E] / [a] [b] [c] [d] [e]
56 [A] [B] [C] [D] [E] / [a] [b] [c] [d] [e]
57 [A] [B] [C] [D] [E] / [a] [b] [c] [d] [e]
58 [A] [B] [C] [D] [E] / [a] [b] [c] [d] [e]
59 [A] [B] [C] [D] [E] / [a] [b] [c] [d] [e]
60 [A] [B] [C] [D] [E] / [a] [b] [c] [d] [e]

Normal Values

NB. These values may vary according to local populations

Haematology
Haemoglobin
Males	13.5–17.5 g/dl
Females	11.5–15.5 g/dl
MCV	76–98 fl
PCV	35–55%
WCC	4–11 × 10⁹/l
Neut.	2.5–7.58 × 10⁹/l
Lymph.	1.5–3.5 × 10⁹/l
Plts	150–400 × 10⁹/l
ESR	0–10mm in the 1st hour
PT	10.6–14.9 s
PTT	23.0–35.0 s
TT	10.5–15.5 s
Fib	125–300 mg/dl
V_{B12}	160–900 pmol/l
Folate	1.5–10.0 × μg/l
Ferritin	
Males	20–250 × μg/l
Females	10–120 × μg/l

Immunoglobulins

IgM	0.5–2.0 g/l
IgG	5–16 g/l
IgA	1.0–4.0 g/l

Biochemistry

Na	135–145 mmol/l
K	3.5–5.0 mmol/l
U	2.5–6.5 mmol/l
Cr	50–120 × μmol/l
ALT	5–30 iu/l
AST	10–40 iu/l
Bili.	2–17 × mmol/l
Alk	P 30–130 iu/l
Alb.	35–55 g/l
γGT	5–30 iu/l
αFP	<10 ku/l
CCa	2.20–2.60 mmol/l
PO_4	0.70–1.40 mmol/l
CK	23–175 iu/l
LDH	100–190 iu/l
Amylase	<200 u/l
Lactate	0.5–2.2 mmol/l
Mg^{2+}	0.75–1.00 mmol/l
Urate	0.1–0.4 mol/l
CRP	0–10 mg/l

Diabetes

Random glucose	3.5–5.5 mmol/l*
*If >5.5 then OGTT 2 hrs:	<7.8 =Normal
	7.8–11 = IGT
	>11.1 = DM
HbA_{1C}	<7.0%

Endocrinology

Prolactin	<400 mu/l
ACTH	<18pmol/l
Cortisol	
0900	200–700 nmol/l
2400	<50 nmol/l
TSH	0.17–3.2 mu/l
T_4	11–22 pmol/l
FSH	
Prepubertal children	<5 u/l
Women	
Follicular phase	2.5–10 u/l
Mid-cycle	25–70 u/l
Luteal phase	0.3–2 u/l
Postmenopausal	>30 u/l
Men	1–8 u/l
LH	
Prepubertal children	<5 u/l
Women	
Follicular phase	2.5–10 u/l
Mid-cycle	25–70 u/l
Luteal phase	0.5–13 u/l
Postmenopausal	>30 u/l
Men	1–10 u/l
Cholesterol	<5.2 mmol/l
Triglycerides	0–1.5 mmol/l
LDL	<3.5 mmol/l
HDL	<1.0 mmol/l
Total/HDL	<5.0 mmol/l

Blood Gases

pH	7.35–7.45
pCO_2	4.6–6.0 kPa
pO_2	10.5–13.5 kPa
HCO_3	24–30 mmol/l
BE	2–2.0 mmol/l

CSF

Protein	< 0.45 g/l
Glucose	2.5 –3.9 mmol/l (two-thirds plasma)
Cells	< 5 (WCC)
Opening Pressure	6–20 cmH$_2$O

Multiple Choice Questions

PAPER 1

Questions (answers, page 15)

---

50 questions: time allowed, 2 hours.
Mark your answers with a tick (True) or a cross (False) in the box provided. Leave the box blank for 'Don't know'. Do not look at the answers until you have completed the whole question paper.

1.1   The following drugs should be given early in acute asthma:

☐   A   oxygen
☐   B   nebulised bronchodilator
☐   C   IV bronchodilator
☐   D   magnesium
☐   E   corticosteroids
☐   F   aminophylline

1.2   Selegiline

☐   A   is a dopamine agonist
☐   B   delays disease progression
☐   C   decreases mortality
☐   D   should only be prescribed once L-dopa therapy has been established
☐   E   reduces end-of-dose deterioration

1

1.3 **The following infections are correctly paired with the appropriate treatment:**

☐ A *Candida* – amphotericin
☐ B *Neisseria meningitidis* – benzylpenicillin
☐ C *Heliobacter pylori* – omeprazole, clarithromycin and metronidazole
☐ D *Mycoplasma* pneumonia – amoxicillin
☐ E *Mycobacterium tuberculosis* – isoniazid, rifampicin and pyrazinamide
☐ F herpes simplex – aciclovir

1.4 **The following statements are true:**

☐ A Clomifene blocks oestrogen receptors
☐ B Octreotide inhibits growth hormone releasing hormone
☐ C Clonidine blocks alpha-2 adrenoreceptors
☐ D Lithium blocks the effects of antidiuretic hormone (ADH) on the kidney
☐ E Sibutramine blocks 5-hydroxytryptamine (5HT) receptors

1.5 **Omeprazole**

☐ A is a recognised treatment for reflux oesophagitis
☐ B causes diarrhoea
☐ C is an antacid
☐ D causes testicular atrophy
☐ E is a recognised cause of gynaecomastia

1.6 **Angiotensin-converting enzyme (ACE) inhibitors**

☐ A are given intravenously for acute left ventricular failure
☐ B may cause first-dose hypotension
☐ C reverse left ventricular hypertrophy
☐ D should not be given with bendroflumethiazide (bendrofluazide)
☐ E prevent myocardial infarction

1.7 Abrupt withdrawal of corticosteroids is considered safe if

- ☐ A treatment has been given for 3–6 weeks
- ☐ B the underlying disease has resolved
- ☐ C there have been repeated short courses (<3 days each)
- ☐ D a patient has received 40 mg prednisolone daily for 2–3 days
- ☐ E a patient has received 10 mg daily for 6 months

1.8 In a double-blind trial

- ☐ A the patient and doctor are blind
- ☐ B no one knows which treatment the patient is receiving
- ☐ C the patient receives the active drug first and then placebo
- ☐ D the patient knows that he is taking part in a trial
- ☐ E the patient must receive a placebo drug

1.9 Tetracycline

- ☐ A can be used topically for acne
- ☐ B is used in exacerbations of chronic pulmonary airways disease
- ☐ C binds to calcium
- ☐ D is teratogenic
- ☐ E may cause renal failure

1.10 Regarding Parkinson's disease

- ☐ A it is due to deficiency of the neurotransmitter dopamine
- ☐ B selegiline is given with L-dopa to reduce end-of-dose deterioration
- ☐ C the treatment of choice is L-dopa with benserazide
- ☐ D it is associated with galactorrhoea
- ☐ E can be treated with antimuscarinic drugs

1.11 The following drugs are paired with their respective antidotes:

☐ A Morphine – Naloxone
☐ B Diazepam – Flumazenil
☐ C Heparin – Warfarin
☐ D Insulin – Glucose
☐ E Iron – Desferrioxamine
☐ F Paracetamol – N-acetylcysteine

1.12 Thiazide diuretics

☐ A cause hypokalaemia
☐ B may cause a rise in plasma urate levels
☐ C may cause hyperglycaemia
☐ D cause first-dose hypotension
☐ E should be given with furosemide (frusemide)

1.13 It is recognised that the following drugs increase the risk of the cancer specified:

☐ A Omeprazole – gastric cancer
☐ B Oestrogens – uterine cancer
☐ C Nicotinic acid – bronchial carcinoma
☐ D Phenytoin – lymphoma
☐ E Cyclophosphamide – testicular tumours

1.14 In a patient who has taken a paracetamol overdose

☐ A treatment includes IV N-acetylcysteine within 24 hours of ingestion
☐ B treatment should include charcoal and methionine
☐ C the patient will be unconscious within 6 hours
☐ D blood levels should be determined 4 hours or more after ingestion
☐ E there is a risk of hepatic damage

1.15 Gastrointestinal bleeding is a recognised unwanted effect of the following drugs:

☐ A Ibuprofen
☐ B Warfarin
☐ C Alcohol
☐ D Prednisolone
☐ E Aspirin
☐ F Paracetamol
☐ G Misoprostol
☐ H Ranitidine
☐ I Omeprazole

1.16 Side-effects of NSAIDs (non-steroidal anti-inflammatory drugs) include

☐ A reversible acute renal failure
☐ B sodium retention and hyperkalaemia
☐ C asthma
☐ D myocardial infarction
☐ E seizures

1.17 Unwanted effects commonly seen with loop diuretics are

☐ A hypokalaemia
☐ B metabolic acidosis
☐ C hypertension
☐ D ototoxicity
☐ E gastrointestinal bleeding

1.18 Hepatotoxicity is a recognised feature of the following drugs:

☐ A Paracetamol
☐ B Halothane
☐ C Rifampicin
☐ D Chlorpromazine
☐ E Methotrexate
☐ F Spironolactone

5

1.19 'Human' insulin

- ☐ A has slower onset of action than equivalent units of conventional insulin
- ☐ B is made from extracts of human pancreas
- ☐ C should not be given during pregnancy
- ☐ D is more expensive than porcine insulin
- ☐ E is more likely than synthetic insulin to cause lipo-atrophy

1.20 Lidocaine (lignocaine) when used as a local anaesthetic

- ☐ A is more effective in inflamed tissue
- ☐ B blocks calcium channels
- ☐ C must be given with adrenaline (epinephrine)
- ☐ D may cause convulsions
- ☐ E is effective within 5 minutes

1.21 Morphine

- ☐ A relieves pain by its action on peripheral opioid receptors
- ☐ B is converted to diamorphine
- ☐ C causes diarrhoea
- ☐ D causes pupil constriction
- ☐ E stimulates the chemoreceptor trigger zone

1.22 A 35-year-old diabetic woman, well controlled on insulin therapy develops a short illness and is admitted semi-conscious. She is ketotic with a serum pH of 7.5, HCO_3 of 14 mmol/l, K^+ 3.5 mmol/l, glucose 30 mmol/l, urea 20 mmol/l. Treatment should include

- ☐ A 1 litre of water orally
- ☐ B half the dose of insulin
- ☐ C 20 units Actrapid® insulin IV immediately
- ☐ D potassium chloride 40 mmol orally
- ☐ E potassium chloride 40 mmol IV in 5 minutes

1.23 The following may precipitate gout:

- ☐ A Prednisolone
- ☐ B Allopurinol
- ☐ C Indometacin
- ☐ D Furosemide (frusemide)
- ☐ E Colchicine

1.24 The following are used to treat atrial fibrillation (AF):

- ☐ A Lidocaine (lignocaine)
- ☐ B Adrenaline (epinephrine)
- ☐ C Digoxin
- ☐ D Verapamil
- ☐ E Warfarin

1.25 Grand mal convulsions are a recognised unwanted effect of

- ☐ A Penicillin
- ☐ B Aminophylline
- ☐ C Lidocaine (lignocaine)
- ☐ D Lithium
- ☐ E Doxapram

1.26 The following have anxiolytic effects:

- ☐ A Chlordiazepoxide
- ☐ B Chlorpropamide
- ☐ C Chlorhexidine
- ☐ D Chlorothiazide
- ☐ E Chlorpromazine
- ☐ F Chloramphenicol

1.27 Recognised treatments of ulcerative colitis include

- ☐ A Sulfasalazine
- ☐ B Omeprazole
- ☐ C Prednisolone enema
- ☐ D Codeine phosphate
- ☐ E Senna

1.28 In the treatment of peptic ulcers

- ☐ A Omeprazole acts as a prostaglandin analogue
- ☐ B Misoprostol may cause constipation
- ☐ C Ranitidine may inhibit liver microsomal enzymes
- ☐ D Sucralfate must be taken with food
- ☐ E Metronidazole may be used

1.29 In anaphylaxis

- ☐ A IV hydrocortisone gives immediate relief
- ☐ B IV penicillin is the treatment of choice
- ☐ C IV adrenaline (epinephrine) should be given promptly
- ☐ D IV chlorphenamine (chlorpheniramine) is indicated
- ☐ E IV salbutamol may be given

1.30 In a trial of stroke prevention, 6% of the patients in the placebo group had strokes and 4% of patients in the 'warfarin' group had strokes. Regarding these figures

- ☐ A the relative risk reduction is 33%
- ☐ B the absolute risk reduction is 2%
- ☐ C there is statistically no significant difference in the results
- ☐ D the number of patients required for treatment to prevent one stroke is 50
- ☐ E the number of strokes prevented for every bleed is 50

1.31 Hormone replacement treatment (HRT)

☐ A   may cause endometrial cancer
☐ B   prevents osteoarthritis
☐ C   reduces the risk of pulmonary embolism
☐ D   increases the risk of breast cancer
☐ E   should be given to all postmenopausal women

1.32 The following are true in relation to pharmacokinetic variation:

☐ A   slow acetylators require larger or more frequent doses of
        isoniazid than fast acetylators to obtain the desired therapeutic
        response
☐ B   patients with glucose-6-phosphate dehydrogenase (G6PD)
        deficiency should avoid aspirin
☐ C   oxidant drugs cause haemolytic anaemia in glutathione
        synthetase deficiency
☐ D   patients with pseudocholinesterase deficiency require an
        increased dose of suxamethonium to obtain the desired
        therapeutic response
☐ E   ingestion of alcohol in patients with accelerated alcohol
        dehydrogenase activity is responsible for extensive
        vasodilation, facial flushing and tachycardia

1.33 The following substances taken in acute overdose are correctly paired with their specific antidote:

☐ A   β-blockers – Glucagon
☐ B   Iron – Desferrioxamine
☐ C   Digoxin – Isoprenaline
☐ D   Diazepam – Naloxone
☐ E   Warfarin – Vitamin K

1.34 The following drugs have an anti-emetic effect:

- ☐ A Metoclopramide
- ☐ B Granisetron
- ☐ C Omeprazole
- ☐ D Cyclizine
- ☐ E Hyoscine

1.35 The following are recognised unwanted effects of the drugs with which they have been paired:

- ☐ A asthma with aspirin
- ☐ B ventricular fibrillation (VF) with lidocaine (lignocaine)
- ☐ C tachycardia with propanolol
- ☐ D bronchospasm with atenolol
- ☐ E bronchospasm with paracetamol

1.36 Diazepam

- ☐ A is addictive
- ☐ B should be withdrawn gradually
- ☐ C acts on the GABA receptor complex
- ☐ D acts on dopamine receptors
- ☐ E may cause insomnia

1.37 Prednisolone may be used to treat

- ☐ A ulcerative colitis
- ☐ B temporal arteritis
- ☐ C acute asthma
- ☐ D appendicitis
- ☐ E acute peptic ulceration

1.38 During cardiopulmonary resuscitation

- [ ] A the intravenous route should be used for drug administration
- [ ] B electromechanical dissociation (EMD) should be treated with atropine
- [ ] C ventricular fibrillation (VF) should be treated with atropine
- [ ] D asystole should be treated with adrenaline (epinephrine)
- [ ] E bicarbonate is essential

1.39 Simvastatin

- [ ] A reduces low-density lipoprotein (LDL) cholesterol by 35%
- [ ] B lowers high-density lipoprotein (HDL) cholesterol
- [ ] C reduces mortality after myocardial infarction
- [ ] D causes drug-induced hepatitis
- [ ] E may cause proximal myopathy

1.40 Aspirin is contraindicated in

- [ ] A young children
- [ ] B acute myocardial infarction
- [ ] C asthma
- [ ] D intermittent claudication
- [ ] E haemorrhagic stroke

1.41 Warfarin

- [ ] A is reversed by vitamin K
- [ ] B is safe in pregnancy
- [ ] C is used to treat deep vein thrombosis
- [ ] D dosage depends on prothrombin time
- [ ] E is metabolised by the liver

1.42 The following skin conditions are paired with their correct treatment:

☐ A herpes simplex – aciclovir cream
☐ B impetigo – metronidazole
☐ C acne – hydrocortisone
☐ D scabies – malathion
☐ E psoriasis – coal tar

1.43 The following are examples of pro-drugs:

☐ A Diamorphine
☐ B Enalapril
☐ C Paracetamol
☐ D Levodopa
☐ E Prednisone

1.44 The following pairs of drugs act on the same receptor:

☐ A Noradrenaline (norepinephrine) and atropine
☐ B Salbutamol and propranolol
☐ C Ipratropium and salmeterol
☐ D Atropine and ondansetron
☐ E Morphine and naloxone

1.45 The following statements are correct:

☐ A alkaline diuresis is useful in the treatment of aspirin overdose
☐ B acid diuresis is useful in the treatment of amfetamine overdose
☐ C probenecid is uricosuric
☐ D morphine is excreted in bile
☐ E digoxin is excreted unchanged in the urine

1.46 The following drugs are hepatic enzyme inducers:

- ☐ A Rifampicin
- ☐ B Cimetidine
- ☐ C Phenytoin
- ☐ D Ranitidine
- ☐ E Carbamazepine

1.47 The following statements regarding antiepileptics are correct:

- ☐ A Sodium vaproate causes gum hypertrophy
- ☐ B Ethosuximide is the drug of choice in absence seizures
- ☐ C Phenytoin is associated with an increased risk of neural tube defects during pregnancy
- ☐ D Gabapentin is used in status epilepticus
- ☐ E Carbamazepine may be used for grand mal seizures

1.48 The following are true of antibiotics used for urinary tract infections (UTIs):

- ☐ A they must be given as a pessary
- ☐ B a 5-day course is required to treat the infection adequately
- ☐ C they must be excreted by the kidney
- ☐ D they should be given after culture and sensitivity results are established
- ☐ E oral trimethoprim is the drug of choice for uncomplicated infection

1.49 Adenosine

- ☐ A is used to terminate ventricular tachycardia
- ☐ B has a very short half-life of 8 seconds
- ☐ C effects are enhanced by theophylline
- ☐ D may cause bronchospasm and therefore should not be used in asthmatics
- ☐ E acts on α-receptors

1.50 Glyceryl trinitrate (GTN)

☐ A is contraindicated in unstable angina
☐ B enhances the release of vascular nitric oxide
☐ C can be given sublingually
☐ D degrades in sunlight
☐ E often causes the development of tolerance
☐ F causes headaches

PAPER 1

Answers

The correct answer options for each question are given below.

1.1	A B E	1.26	A
1.2	E	1.27	A C D
1.3	A B C E F	1.28	E
1.4	A B D	1.29	D E
1.5	A B E	1.30	A B D
1.6	B C E	1.31	A D
1.7	D	1.32	B C E
1.8	D	1.33	A B E
1.9	A B C D E	1.34	A B D E
1.10	A B C E	1.35	A D
1.11	A B D E F	1.36	A B C
1.12	A B C	1.37	A B C
1.13	B D E	1.38	A D
1.14	A D E	1.39	A C D E
1.15	A B C D E	1.40	A C E
1.16	A B C E	1.41	A C D E
1.17	A D	1.42	A D E
1.18	A B C D E F	1.43	B D E
1.19	All false	1.44	B E
1.20	D E	1.45	A B C D E
1.21	D E	1.46	A C E
1.22	All false	1.47	B C E
1.23	B D	1.48	E
1.24	C D	1.49	B
1.25	A B C D E	1.50	B C D E F

MCQs

Paper 1

Answers and teaching notes

1.1 Acute asthma   Answers: A B E

The key word in this question is 'early'. High concentrations of oxygen should be given, at a flow rate of 6l/min, as patients are likely to have a low PaO$_2$. Nebulised bronchodilators such as salbutamol should be started immediately. If there is no improvement the dose is repeated at 15-minute intervals. Intravenous bronchodilators are only given to patients who fail to respond to nebulised bronchodilators. Cortico-steroids should be given either orally or intravenously as soon as possible, although the benefit may not be seen until after about 6 hours. Magnesium should be reserved for patients who fail to respond to a nebulised bronchodilator. Aminophylline is only rarely given in acute asthma because of its side-effects and limited efficacy.

1.2 Selegiline   Answer: E

Selegiline is a monoamine-oxidase-B inhibitor. It has been used to reduce end-of-dose deterioration but more recently it has been found to delay the need for L-dopa therapy if started early. However, it has been suggested that there is an increase in mortality when selegiline is used with L-dopa.

1.3 Infections   Answers: A B C E F

Amphotericin is a macrolide antibiotic that has poor oral absorption and is therefore used to treat fungal infections of the gastrointestinal tract. It is given intravenously for systemic infections, but renal toxicity is a major side-effect. Penicillins are active against most

Gram-positive and Gram-negative bacteria, and intravenous benzyl-penicillin is used to treat bacterial meningitis. Minocycline is an example of a tetracycline that is effective against *N. meningitidis* but does **not** cross the blood–brain barrier and is therefore not used to treat meningitis. *H. pylori* infection is implicated in peptic ulcer disease and combination therapy with at least three drugs is used for eradication; other examples include omeprazole, amoxicillin and metronidazole, or omeprazole, clarithromycin, metronidazole and bismuth. Tetracyclines are the drug of choice for mycoplasma as well as rickettsial and chlamydial infection. Penicillins are ineffective because mycoplasma do not have a bacterial cell wall. Mycobacterial infections cause tuberculosis or leprosy. *M. tuberculosis* is treated with isoniazid, rifampicin and pyrazinamide for 2 months, then isoniazid and rifampicin for 4 months. *M. leprae* is treated with dapsone and rifampicin. Herpes simplex causes cold sores, ulcers and mouth infections and is treated with aciclovir.

1.4   Correct statements   **Answers: A B D**

Clomifene blocks oestrogen receptors in the hypothalamus, resulting in gonadotrophin release. It is used in the treatment of female infertility. Octreotide and lantreotide are analogues of somatostatin, which inhibits hormone release by the hypothalamus. Somatostatin is generally known as a 'blocker'. Clonidine is a centrally acting antihypertensive. Prazosin and doxazosin are alpha adrenoceptor blocking drugs used in the treatment of hypertension. Lithium is excreted by the kidney. Its renal effects include polyuria resulting from inhibition of ADH. There is also sodium retention due to increased aldosterone release. Renal tubular damage can occur and renal function should be monitored. Lithium effects are increased in sodium depletion. Other side effects are nausea, vomiting, weight gain, hypothyroidism and tremor.

1.5   Omeprazole   **Answers: A B E**

Omeprazole irreversibly inhibits the hydrogen/potassium-ATPase (proton pump) system, thereby reducing gastric acid secretion. Omeprazole can be used to treat peptic ulcer disease (especially when resistant to H_2-receptor antagonist treatment), reflux oesophagitis, Zollinger–Ellison syndrome, and *H. pylori* infection as part of triple therapy. Side-effects are uncommon and include rash, diarrhoea, dizziness, headache, impotence, gynaecomastia and confusion. It is not an antacid – antacids work by neutralising gastric acid.

1.6 Angiotensin-converting enzyme (ACE) inhibitors   Answers: B C E

ACE inhibitors are given orally, and often cause first-dose hypotension and postural hypotension. Intravenous administration is associated with severe hypotension. ACE inhibitors reverse LV hypertrophy in hypertension, more effectively than other antihypertensive drugs. Diuretic treatment, hyponatraemia, or extracellular fluid depletion increase the risk of ACE-inhibitor-induced hypotension. Therefore, ACE inhibitors and diuretics should be combined with great care. ACE inhibitors reduce the risk of myocardial infarction (MI) in 'secondary prevention', that is treatment of high-risk groups, including patients with diabetes, previous MI, or hypertension.

1.7 Abrupt withdrawal of corticosteroids   Answer: D

The Committee on Safety of Medicines has recommended that gradual withdrawal of systemic corticosteroids should be considered in patients whose disease is unlikely to relapse and have received more than three weeks' treatment, received more than 40 mg prednisolone daily, recently received repeated courses, had a short course within 1 year of stopping long-term therapy, been given repeat doses in the evening, or if there are other possible causes of adrenal suppression. During corticosteroid withdrawal the dose may be rapidly lowered to physiological doses (i.e. 7–15 mg daily) and then more gradually. Assessment may be required to ensure that disease relapse does not occur during withdrawal.

1.8 A double-blind trial   Answer: D

Study volunteers must give informed consent to take part in a trial, and will be aware that they are taking part in a trial. In a double-blind trial, the administering doctor and volunteer/patient do not know what treatment is being administered, so as to minimise subjective bias. It may be the test drug or the placebo/active comparator drug. A third party controls the administration of drug. In a single-blind trial, the administering doctor knows what the patient is receiving but the patient does not. In a crossover trial, the patient receives both treatments, each for a set period of time. It is obvious that the patient does not necessarily receive a placebo drug.

1.9   Tetracycline   **Answers: A B C D E**

Tetracycline can be used topically (for acne or rosacea) or given orally for systemic infections. It is a broad-spectrum antibiotic and is used to treat: chlamydia, rickettsia, brucella, *Borrelia burgdorferi*, mycoplasma infections and *Haemophilus influenzae*. It is used in chronic bronchitis to treat *H. influenzae* infection. Tetracycline is chelated by calcium and incorporated into growing bones and teeth: this can cause yellow discoloration and dental hypoplasia. It should not be given to pregnant or breast-feeding women or to children under 12 years. It has a catabolic effect, causing a rise in plasma urea and is excreted in the urine. It can cause renal failure.

1.10 Parkinson's disease   **Answers: A B C E**

Progressive degeneration in the substantia nigra causes a relative deficiency of dopamine (DA). Selegiline is a monoamine-oxidase-B inhibitor and is given with L-dopa (the precursor of DA) to reduce end-of-dose effects. Benserazide is a peripheral dopa-decarboxylase inhibitor, which prevents conversion of L-dopa to dopamine in the circulation, so that more L-dopa crosses the blood–brain barrier. DA deficiency is limited to the substantia nigra and, therefore, prolactin production by the pituitary remains normal. Antimuscarinic drugs correct the relative excess of cholinergic activity (compared to dopaminergic activity), and are particularly useful for treating tremor and rigidity in parkinsonism.

1.11 Drugs paired with their respective antidotes   **Answers: A B D E F**

Antidotes are useful in some cases of drug toxicity. Opioids can cause coma and cardiorespiratory depression, and naloxone is a useful opioid-receptor antagonist. However, it has a short duration of action and, therefore, continuous naloxone infusion or repeated administration is often required. Flumazenil is a benzodiazepine antagonist, and is a particularly effective antidote for midazolam. It also has a short half-life, so its effects must be monitored closely. Heparin and warfarin both increase clotting time. Glucose is often used to correct the hypo-glycaemia resulting from insulin overdosage; glucagon can be used to directly oppose the effects of insulin. Desferrioxamine chelates heavy metals and enhances the clearance of iron. N-acetylcysteine is the treatment of choice in paracetamol overdosage to prevent glutathione depletion. Methionine can also be used in addition to N-acetylcysteine, but is of debatable importance.

1.12 Thiazide diuretics   Answers: A B C

Thiazides are very commonly used and therefore it is important to know their indications and side-effects. Thiazides inhibit sodium reabsorption and cause a diuresis, causing a loss of Na^+ with water. They are used in the treatment of hypertension and congestive cardiac failure. Metabolic side-effects include alkalosis, hyponatraemia, hypokalaemia, hypomagnesaemia, hypercalcaemia, hyperglycaemia, hyperuricaemia and hypertriglyceridaemia. They may cause hypochloraemic alkalosis. Other side-effects include gastrointestinal disturbance, impotence, photosensitivity, neutropenia, thrombocytopenia and pancreatitis. First-dose hypotension occurs with ACE inhibitors or α-blockers. Furosemide (frusemide) is a potent loop diuretic and is usually not given in combination with a thiazide.

1.13 Drugs recognised as increasing the risk of the cancer specified
Answers: B D E

The presence of *Helicobacter pylori* is a risk factor for gastric cancer, while eradication therapy includes treatment with omeprazole or other proton pump inhibitor. Early animal studies suggested an increased risk of gastric cancer, but this has not been seen in humans. Some tumours are hormone-dependent, e.g.

- breast cancer – oestrogens
- prostate cancer – androgens
- uterine cancer – oestrogens

Nicotine, a constituent of tobacco smoke, has been implicated in the development of lung cancer. Phenytoin causes numerous blood dyscrasias, and lymphoma has been reported. Cyclophosphamide is used to treat chronic lymphocytic leukaemia, lymphomas and solid tumours. Side-effects include bone marrow suppression, alopecia, testicular damage, increased acute non-lymphocytic leukaemia.

1.14 Paracetamol overdose   Answers: A D E

Toxic doses of paracetamol cause early nausea and vomiting. After 24–48 hours, liver damage occurs and renal tubular necrosis may also occur due to glutathione depletion. Overdose treatment is gastric lavage, oral activated charcoal, N-acetylcysteine IV and/or methionine orally. Plasma paracetamol concentration measured 4 hours after ingestion is a strong prognostic indicator, and patients at highest risk of liver damage can be identified and treated. N-acetyl-cysteine protects the liver if given within 24 hours of ingestion, whereas oral methionine should be given within 12 hours.

1.15 Gastrointestinal (GI) bleeding   Answers: A B C D E

NSAIDs and aspirin cause gastric irritation and peptic ulceration. Corticosteroids confer an increased risk of peptic ulceration, particularly in combination with a NSAID or aspirin. The anticoagulant effect of warfarin causes GI blood loss due to the normal sloughing of epithelial cells. Alcohol causes acute erosive gastritis; in alcohol-induced liver damage with portal hypertension, there may also be blood loss from oesophageal varices. It is worth knowing drugs that cause and prevent GI bleeding. Paracetamol does not irritate the gastric mucosa. Misoprostol is a prostaglandin analogue that enhances bicarbonate secretion and promotes peptic ulcer healing. Ranitidine is an H_2-receptor antagonist, and omeprazole is a proton pump inhibitor; both reduce gastric acid secretion and promote ulcer healing.

21

1.16 Side-effects of NSAIDs   Answers: A B C E

Renal failure may occur, especially in patients with pre-existing renal impairment. This is reversible if the drug if stopped early. GI disturbance includes ulceration and bleeding. NSAIDs inhibit prostaglandin synthesis. They indirectly suppress renin and aldosterone secretion which results in hyperkalaemia and Na^+ retention. Hypersensitivity reactions include rashes, bronchospasm and tinnitus. NSAIDs do not increase the risk of myocardial infarction, but aggravate hypertension and cardiac failure due to increased fluid retention. NSAIDs can cause seizures, particularly in neonates or in overdose; treatment is with diazepam.

1.17 Unwanted effects commonly seen with loop diuretics
Answers: A D

K^+ loss and ototoxicity are unwanted effects commonly seen with loop diuretics, in addition to hypotension, hypocalcaemia, hypomagnesaemia, and metabolic alkalosis. The risk of ototoxicity is greatest if large doses are given by intravenous bolus administration, and risk is increased when given with aminoglycosides. Loop diuretics are powerful diuretics and can be used to treat hypertension. GI disturbance is very rare.

1.18 Hepatotoxicity   Answers: A B C D E F

Paracetamol is especially hepatotoxic in overdose. Halothane is a volatile liquid anaesthetic that causes severe hepatitis. Liver function should be monitored whilst taking rifampicin, and the dose should be reduced in hepatic impairment. Chlorpromazine causes reversible cholestatic jaundice. Long-term methotrexate treatment causes irreversible hepatic fibrosis. Spironolactone can cause hepatoxicity, although it is often used to treat oedema and ascites in liver cirrhosis.

1.19 'Human' insulin   Answers: All false

Human sequence insulin preparations tend to have a more rapid onset of action and shorter duration of action. Human insulin is produced by enzymatic modification of porcine insulin or synthesised by recombinant technology using *Escherichia coli.*

Human insulin is safe in pregnancy. Preparations vary and some 'human' insulins are cheaper than porcine and bovine preparations. Insulin is inactivated in the gastrointestinal tract and must therefore be given by injection, usually subcutaneous. Lipo-atrophy is an immune-mediated response that is more common with synthetic insulin, and minimised by changing injection site.

1.20 Lidocaine (lignocaine)   Answers: D E

Inflamed tissues are often acidotic, resulting in high ionisation of local anaesthetic. This makes it less able to permeate the cell membrane. In alkaline pH, non-ionised molecules permeate the cell membrane more easily. Local anaesthetics block sodium channels and, therefore, prevent nerve conduction. Epinephrine (adrenaline) causes vasoconstriction, which prolongs the action of local anaesthetic, but it is not necessary. Lidocaine (lignocaine) can cause tremor, agitation and convulsions; these can occur following systemic administration, or where excessive local use causes a systemic effect. It is effective within 5 minutes, and has a variable duration of action depending on how quickly the drug is removed from the tissue. Skin preparations, e.g. Emla® cream, may take longer to penetrate to the site of action than local drug injection.

1.21 Morphine   Answers: D E

Morphine acts as an opioid-receptor agonist in the brain and spinal cord, rather than peripheral sites. Diamorphine is metabolised to morphine, and morphine is conjugated in the liver to morphine-6-glucuronide, which is itself a potent analgesic. Pinpoint pupils are seen, particularly in overdosage.The chemoreceptor trigger zone is stimulated, causing nausea and vomiting as side-effects, and it is often given with an anti-emetic. Constipation is a well-known side-effect.

1.22 A 35-year-old diabetic woman   Answers: All false

This lady is in diabetic ketoacidosis. Normal saline should be given

IV to replace fluid. Insulin is given by IV infusion pump. IV infusion is commenced at 6 units/h. If IV administration is not possible, 20 units is given IM followed by 6 units IM every hour. KCl should be added to the infusion of sodium chloride. Potassium chloride 40 mmol IV in 5 minutes is too rapid. KCl is simply added to the infusion to prevent hypokalaemia induced by insulin.

1.23 Gout   Answers: B D

Acute gout consists of acute arthritis produced by inflammation of urate crystals that have been deposited in synovial joints. There is often a good response to corticosteroids due to their anti-inflammatory properties. Allopurinol inhibits uric acid synthesis by inhibition of xanthine oxidase. It is used in the long-term treatment of gout, but sudden lowering of urate concentrations can precipitate an acute attack. NSAIDs are used for their analgesic and anti-inflammatory effects in the acute attack. Furosemide (frusemide) can cause dehydration with precipitation of urate crystals in joints. Colchicine is used to prevent gout or to treat acute attacks.

1.24 Atrial fibrillation   Answers: C D

Lidocaine (lignocaine) acts on ventricular arrhythmias. Epinephrine (adrenaline) predisposes to atrial fibrillation; adenosine is used to terminate supraventricular tachycardia (SVT) but it has a short half-life. Digoxin and verapamil block the atrioventricular (AV) node and slow the ventricular rate. Warfarin is given to prevent embolisation, rather than treat atrial fibrillation itself.

1.25 Grand mal convulsions   Answers: A B C D E

Any of the penicillins can cause fits, especially in renal failure and in high doses. Aminophylline is no longer a first-line drug in the treatment of acute asthma; it has many side-effects, including convulsions and arrhythmia. Lidocaine (lignocaine) decreases the threshold for convulsions. Doxapram is a respiratory stimulant that may also cause fits.

1.26 Anxiolytic effects   Answer: A

These drugs have similar names and are easily confused. Chlordiazepoxide has anxiolytic effects. It is a benzodiazepine. Chlorpropamide is a sulphonylurea used in the treatment of diabetes mellitus. Chlorhexidine is an antiseptic. Chlorothiazide is a thiazide diuretic. Chlorpromazine is an antipsychotic. Chloramphenicol is an antibiotic.

1.27 Recognised treatments of ulcerative colitis   Answers: A C D

Sulfasalazine is sulfapyridine combined with 5-aminosalicylic acid. It is used to prevent acute attacks of colitis. Omeprazole is a proton pump inhibitor effective in reducing gastric acid secretion. Prednisolone enema is given locally for its anti-inflammatory effects, while more severe disease requires systemic treatment. Colitis results in watery diarrhoea, which can be symptomatically controlled with codeine in mild cases. Opiates increase the risk of toxic megacolon and sepsis. Laxatives facilitate bowel movement in proctitis but bulking agents are more useful than irritants like senna.

1.28 The treatment of peptic ulcers   Answer: E

Omeprazole is a proton pump inhibitor. Misoprostol is a prostaglandin analogue and has protective properties in peptic ulceration. Side-effects are diarrhoea, nausea and vomiting, dyspepsia and abnormal vaginal bleeding. Ranitidine (an H_2-receptor antagonist) inhibits hepatic drug metabolism by binding to microsomal cytochrome P450. It should therefore be avoided in patients taking warfarin and phenytoin. Sucralfate protects gastric and duodenal mucosa, and should be taken 1 hour before meals. Metronidazole may be used in triple therapy (e.g. with amoxicillin and omeprazole) in eradication of *H. pylori*.

1.29 Anaphylaxis   Answers: D E

Hydrocortisone takes 6 hours to have an effect (100–300 mg). It should be given early to prevent deterioration. Penicillin is often implicated as a cause of anaphylaxis. In anaphylaxis, patients have signs of shock, but antibiotics do not have any role in management. Epinephrine (adrenaline) is given, but the intramuscular route is preferred. Intravenous chlorphenamine (chlorpheniramine) is given after adrenaline (ephinephrine), and continued for 24 to 48 hours to prevent relapse. Patients on β-blockers may not respond adequately to adrenaline (epinephrine), in which case IV salbutamol may be required.

1.30 Stroke prevention   Answers: A B D

There is a 2% decrease with warfarin relative to the placebo and $2/6 = 1/3$. The real difference in number of strokes is $6\% - 4\% = 2\%$. The statistical comparison between the two groups will take account of the numbers in each group. A statistically significant result is seen at p value (not an event rate) of 5% or less. Placebo $\rightarrow$ 6 out of 100 strokes. Warfarin $\rightarrow$ 4 out of 100 stokes. Therefore, 2 out of 100 patients benefit from stroke prevention on warfarin, or 1 in 50. There is no indication of the number of bleeds.

1.31 HRT   Answers: A D

Long-term hormone replacement therapy is most favourable for women without a uterus as oestrogen confers the beneficial effects. However, it cannot be given without progesterone because of an increased risk of uterine cancer. Progesterone may blunt the effect of low-dose oestrogen against myocardial infarction and stroke. There is a definite reduction in osteoporosis (not osteoarthritis), and there is an increased incidence of venous thromboembolism. There is an increased risk of breast cancer that is related to duration of use. This risk disappears within about 5 years of stopping. Breast cancers in HRT users are less likely to have metastatic spread than in non-users. In non-users of HRT who are 50 years old, the incidence of breast cancer developing over the next 20 years is 45 per 1,000. In women using HRT for 5 years, this figure rises by two extra cases per 1,000; 10 years, six extra cases per 1,000; and 15 years, 12 extra cases per 1,000.

1.32 Pharmacokinetic variation: Answers: B C E

In about 50% of the population, drug inactivation by hepatic N-acetyltransferase is slow. Such people (slow acetylators) require a longer time to metabolise drugs that are acetylated and are therefore more susceptible to adverse effects of such drugs (e.g. peripheral neuritis with isoniazid, SLE with hydralazine or procainamide). In the rest of the population, acetylation is rapid. Compared with slow acetylators, they require larger or more frequent doses of drugs that are acetylated (e.g. isoniazid) to obtain the desired therapeutic response.

G6PD is essential for red blood cell (RBC) reduction reactions that maintain cytoskeletal integrity. Patients with G6PD deficiency (which occurs in about 10% of black males) are at increased risk of developing haemolytic anemia when given oxidant drugs, such as antimalarials (e.g. chloroquine or primaquine), aspirin and vitamin K. In patients with RBC glutathione synthetase deficiency (which is similar to but much rarer than G6PD deficiency), oxidant drugs also cause haemolytic anemia. Patients with low levels of RBC glutathione synthetase in hepatocytes are at increased risk of liver damage if given drugs as paracetamol and nitrofurantoin.

About 1 in 1,500 people has plasma pseudocholinesterase deficiency, which delays suxamethonium inactivation. When conventional doses of the drug are given, prolonged paralysis of the respiratory muscles results.

In about 85% of Asian populations and in 5% to 10% of the caucasian, alcohol dehydrogenase (an enzyme involved in ethanol metabolism) operates about five times faster than normal. When such persons ingest alcohol, acetaldehyde accumulates, resulting in extensive vasodilation, facial flushing, and compensatory tachycardia.

1.33 Acute overdose Answers: A B E

Bradycardia and hypotension induced by beta-blocker overdose may respond to intravenous or intramuscular glucagon. Cardiac pacing may be indicated in severe cases.

IV desferrioxamine is used in severe cases of iron poisoning. Treatment should be limited to 24 hours, when exchange transfusion should be considered.

Digoxin overdose resulting in severe bradycardias may be treated with Digibind®. There is no place for positive inotropes or chronotropes.

Benzodiazepine overdose can be reversed with flumazenil although caution must be taken as treatment can provoke seizures, particularly if there is concurrent tricyclic antidepressant use. Warfarin overdose with haemorrhage is treated by omitting further doses of warfarin, giving vitamin K 5 mg IV and giving fresh frozen plasma (or prothrombin complex concentrate of factor II, VII, IX, X).

1.34 Anti-emetic drugs   Answers A B D E

Anti-emetic drugs can be classified according to their mode of action. Antihistamines (e.g. cyclizine) and phenothiazines (e.g. chlorperazine and chlorpromazine) act centrally by inhibiting the chemoreceptor trigger zone (CTZ). They are very effective in the management of nausea occurring with cytotoxic therapy. Domperidone and metoclopramide are dopamine antagonists acting at the CTZ. Metoclopramide also increases gastric motility, thereby reducing gastric distension. Dexamethasone may also be used in vomiting associated with chemotherapy. Hyoscine is an antimuscarinic drug used in motion sickness and has an anti-emetic effect. Omeprazole is a proton pump inhibitor that reduces gastric acid secretion, but does not have anti-emetic properties.

1.35 Unwanted effects   Answers: A D

Aspirin causes gastrointestinal irritation, prolongs bleeding time and may cause bronchospasm and urticaria. Lidocaine (lignocaine) can be used to treat VF and increases myocardial stability. Propanolol is a β-blocker and causes bradycardia. β-blockers may precipitate asthma or bronchospasm. Atenolol is a cardioselective β_1-blocker that has less effect on pulmonary β_2 receptors that mediate bronchospasm. Bronchospasm may occur with non-steroidal anti-inflammatory drugs, but not with paracetamol.

1.36 Diazepam   Answers: A B C

Diazepam (Valium®) is a benzodiazepine used to treat anxiety disorders. It has a prolonged action and is indicated for the short-term treatment of severe anxiety. It should be given for 2 to 4 weeks. Dependence and tolerance occur so the drug should be withdrawn gradually in reducing doses. Benzodiazepines act on receptors that are associated with GABA receptors. Dosage at night may have a hangover effect and affects ability to drive. Paradoxically, aggression may occur while taking benzodiazepines. Withdrawal may cause insomnia, anxiety, tremor and sweating.

1.37 Prednisolone   Answers: A B C

Prednisolone is a glucocorticoid (steroidal) anti-inflammatory drug. It also suppresses allergic reactions, and can be used to treat Crohn's disease, ulcerative colitis, iritis and scleritis, temporal arteritis, vasculitis, acute asthma, rheumatoid arthritis, and cerebral oedema. Corticosteroids may cause peptic ulceration and perforation, particularly in combination with NSAIDs. Corticosteroids can mask the signs of inflammation, resulting in late presentation of acute appendicitis. Other important side-effects are osteoporosis, adrenal suppression, Cushing's syndrome, hyperglycaemia, immunosuppression, neuropsychiatric effects, glaucoma, impaired healing, skin atrophy with striae and bruising.

1.38 Cardiopulmonary resuscitation   Answers: A D

Intravenous access is required to deliver drugs quickly and efficiently. EMD is treated with adrenaline (epinephrine), and the underlying cause should be treated, where possible. VF should be treated by defibrillation and intravenous adrenaline (epinephrine), repeated every 3 minutes if necessary. Asystole is treated with intravenous adrenaline (epinephrine), whereas atropine is used for profound bradycardia. Sodium bicarbonate should only be used with extreme caution, because systemic administration can exacerbate intracellular acidosis.

29

1.39 Simvastatin   Answers: A C D E

The 'statins' inhibit 3-hydroxy-3-methylglutaryl coenzyme A (HGM-CoA) reductase, which is the rate-limiting enzyme in cholesterol synthesis. They lower LDL cholesterol, lower total cholesterol, increase HDL cholesterol, decrease triglycerides, and increase hepatic expression of LDL receptors. The Scandinavian Simvastatin Survival Study showed that simvastatin 20–40 mg caused a 35% reduction in LDL cholesterol and a 30% reduction in cardiovascular mortality. Unwanted effects include gastrointestinal disturbance, insomnia and rash, myositis, hepatitis and angio-oedema. Therefore, serum creatinine kinase and liver biochemistry require monitoring.

1.40 Aspirin   Answers: A C E

Aspirin is contraindicated in children and in breast-feeding due to the risk of Reye's syndrome. It is also contraindicated in peptic ulceration, bleeding disorders, and gout, because it can aggravate these conditions. Aspirin is contraindicated in patients with hypersensitivity to aspirin or NSAIDs, and in asthmatics as it may precipitate an asthma attack. Aspirin and NSAIDs can provoke bronchospasm in non-asthmatic individuals. Low-dose aspirin is used for its antiplatelet action in intermittent claudication and for cerebral prevention of thrombosis. It is given after ischaemic stroke, but not after haemorrhagic stroke unless there is another compelling indication. It is also given after coronary artery bypass graft surgery.

1.41 Warfarin   Answers: A C D E

Warfarin inhibits the reduction of vitamin K, which is required for synthesis of clotting factors II, VII, IX and X. Oral anticoagulants are teratogenic and should be avoided especially in the first trimester; they should also be avoided in the third trimester due to the increased risk of antepartum haemorrhage. Warfarin is used to prevent and treat deep vein thrombosis, pulmonary embolism, atrial fibrillation and patients with prosthetic heart valves. The effect is monitored by prothrombin time, expressed as the international normalised ratio (INR). Warfarin is metabolised by the liver, and has important interactions with hepatic enzyme inhibitors and inducers.

1.42 Skin conditions
Answers: A D E

Aciclovir is used for varicella-zoster (shingles) and herpes simplex skin infections (including genital herpes). Impetigo can be treated by topical fusidic acid or mupirocin, or oral flucloxacillin or erythromycin. Acne can be treated with oral antibiotics, including doxycycline or erythromycin. Malathion or permethrin can be used to treat scabies infestation, and coal tar is used to treat psoriasis and chronic atopic eczema.

1.43 Pro-drugs
Answers: B D E

Diamorphine has some opiate activity, and is converted to morphine by hepatic metabolism. A pro-drug is not active in its parent form, which is why diamorphine is not classified as a pro-drug. Enalapril is converted by hepatic metabolism to enalaprilat, its active form. Paracetamol is converted to toxic metabolites. L-dopa (precursor) is metabolised to dopamine by dopa decarboxylase. Prednisone is converted to prednisolone, which is active.

1.44 Drugs acting on the same receptor
Answers: B E

Noradrenaline (norepinephrine) stimulates adrenergic receptors and atropine blocks muscarinic receptors; salbutamol is a β_2-receptor agonist and propranolol is a β_1-receptor antagonist although they are not entirely receptor type selective; ipratropium is an antimuscarinic bronchodilator whereas salmeterol is a β_2 agonist bronchodilator. Morphine and naloxone both act on opiate receptors; ondansetron acts on $5HT_3$ receptors.

1.45 Correct statements
Answers: A B C D E

Changes in urinary pH can be used to alter drug excretion. Urinary alkalinisation causes weakly acidic drugs to be highly ionised and, therefore, poorly reabsorbed so that clearance is enhanced. Bicarbonate increases urinary pH and increases salicylate elimination. Urinary acidification accelerates the excretion of weakly basic drugs. Probenecid inhibits reabsorption of urate in distal renal tubules and is, therefore, uricosuric. Drugs excreted in bile are broken down in the gut and reabsorbed by the enterohepatic circulation, e.g. morphine. Digoxin is water soluble and the majority is cleared by renal excretion; this is in contrast to digitoxin, which is lipid soluble and cleared by hepatic metabolism.

1.46 Hepatic enzyme inducers   Answers: A C E

A number of drugs act as important enzyme inducers and inhibitors:

Inducers	*Inhibitors*
Phenobarbitone	Cimetidine
Rifampicin	Metrondazole
Ethanol	Chlorpromazine
Carbamazepine	Ciprofloxacin
Griseofulvin	
Phenytoin	

Enzyme inducers increase drug metabolism and reduce drug effects; for example, rifampicin reduces the effectiveness of the oral contraceptive pill. Conversely, enzyme inhibitors delay drug metabolism and enhance drug effects; for example, ciprofloxacin inhibits the metabolism of theophylline and predisposes to toxicity. Learn a list of each of these.

1.47 Antiepileptics   Answers: B C E

Phenytoin causes gingival hypertrophy, peripheral neuropathy, ataxia, nystagmus, rashes, acne, hirsutism, hepatitis, lupus erythematosus, megaloblastic anaemia, agranulocytosis, leucopenia, reduced calcium with rickets/osteomalacia. Ethosuximide and valproate can be used for absence seizures. Phenytoin, carbamazepine and valproate are all teratogenic. The risk of neural tube defects may be reduced by early folate supplementation. In status epilepticus, a number of drugs can be used: intravenous diazepam (or clonazepam or lorazepam), phenytoin or clomethiazole, or rectal paraldehyde. Carbamazepine, phenytoin or valproate may be used to treat grand mal seizures.

1.48 Urinary tract infections   Answer: E

UTIs are treated with the appropriate antibiotic, which can be given orally or intravenously or as a pessary. It is acceptable to give a 3-day course to treat uncomplicated infections. Alternatively, a single large dose may be used. Excretion by the kidney is not compulsory. UTIs are often treated empirically as prompt treatment is required, while awaiting definitive culture results. Trimethoprim or ampicillin can be used, although resistance is increasing.

1.49 Adenosine   Answer: B

Adenosine is used to treat paroxysmal supraventricular tachycardia. It has a half-life of 8–10 seconds. Important side-effects include facial flushing, bronchospasm, nausea and bradycardia, and it should be used with caution in asthmatics. Theophylline is an adenosine antagonist, whereas the effects of adenosine are prolonged by dipyridamole. Adenosine acts on A1, A2 and A3 receptor subtypes.

1.50 Glyceryl trinitrate   Answers: B C D E F

Organic nitrates are vasodilators, increasing coronary flow and thereby reducing pain due to cardiac ischaemia. It is useful in 'stable' and unstable angina. Organic nitrates are metabolised by endothelium to release nitric oxide, which increases with cyclic GMP (cGMP) formation and dephosphorylation of smooth muscle protein to cause vascular smooth muscle relaxation and vasodilatation. Glyceryl trinitrate can be given intravenously, sublingually or transdermally; it cannot be given orally due to extensive first-pass metabolism. GTN is packaged in light-proof containers. Tolerance occurs with the use of longer-acting nitrates such as Ismo®, and to a lesser extent with short-acting nitrates such as GTN. The main side-effects are hypotension and headaches, and tolerance to these effects also occurs.

Multiple Choice Questions

PAPER 2

Questions (answers, page 48)

50 questions: time allowed, 2 hours.
Mark your answers with a tick (True) or a cross (False) in the box provided. Leave the box blank for 'Don't know'. Do not look at the answers until you have completed the whole question paper.

2.1   The major contraindications to thrombolysis are

☐   A   suspected aortic dissection
☐   B   pregnancy
☐   C   warfarin therapy
☐   D   cavitating pulmonary tuberculosis
☐   E   tooth extraction or minor surgery within the last month

2.2   The following are paired with recognised side-effects:

☐   A   Thiazide diuretics (e.g. bendroflumethiazide (bendrofluazide)) and hyperkalaemia
☐   B   Amiodarone and photosensitivity
☐   C   Bromocriptine and hyperprolactinaemia
☐   D   NSAIDs and renal impairment
☐   E   Furosemide (frusemide) and hyperkalaemia

2.3   In an adult male, the following supplements would always be required after pituitary ablation:

☐   A   Insulin
☐   B   Hydrocortisone
☐   C   Fludrocortisone
☐   D   Thyroxine
☐   E   Aldosterone

2.4   The following drugs have been shown to reduce mortality following myocardial infarction (MI):

☐   A   Atenolol
☐   B   Captopril
☐   C   GTN
☐   D   Aspirin
☐   E   Furosemide (frusemide)

2.5   The following are recognised treatments for *Clostridium difficile:*

☐   A   Omeprazole
☐   B   Metronidazole
☐   C   Oral vancomycin
☐   D   Cefuroxime
☐   E   Penicillin

2.6   Digoxin

☐   A   is cleared by the liver
☐   B   should not be given with furosemide (frusemide)
☐   C   is used to treat atrial fibrillation
☐   D   effects are increased by hypokalaemia
☐   E   causes cardiac arrhythmias

2.7 Therapeutic drug monitoring (TDM) is used with the following drugs:

☐ A Nifedipine
☐ B Ciclosporin
☐ C Warfarin
☐ D Gentamicin
☐ E Theophylline

2.8 Metronidazole

☐ A must be given intravenously
☐ B is used to treat *Giardia lamblia*
☐ C should only be used after susceptible organisms have been isolated
☐ D should not be taken with alcohol
☐ E is used in the treatment of pseudomembranous colitis

2.9 A 43-year-old man is given suxamethonium for hernia repair. The following statements are true:

☐ A suxamethonium is a non-depolarising neuromuscular blocker
☐ B prolonged paralysis may occur
☐ C neostigmine is used to reverse the effect
☐ D he may complain of muscle pain after surgery
☐ E atropine may be required

2.10 The following drugs are nephrotoxic:

☐ A Gentamicin
☐ B Furosemide (frusemide)
☐ C Diclofenac
☐ D Amoxicillin
☐ E Ciclosporin

2.11 Lidocaine (lignocaine)

☐ A is metabolised by the liver
☐ B is used for ventricular arrhythmias
☐ C penetrates mucosal membranes
☐ D relieves pain by blocking nociceptors
☐ E causes impaired proprioception before decreasing pain

2.12 Morphine

☐ A is used in the management of myocardial infarction (MI)
☐ B is the analgesic of choice for biliary colic
☐ C causes respiratory depression and suppression of cough
☐ D can be used for post-operative pain in an infusion pump with on-demand boluses operated by the patient
☐ E helps reduce nausea through effects on the chemoreceptor trigger zone

2.13 An adult male is admitted in status epilepticus. The following early treatment is appropriate:

☐ A diazepam *per rectum*
☐ B establish an airway and administer oxygen 60%
☐ C intramuscular phenytoin
☐ D clomethiazole
☐ E flumazenil

2.14 Mesalazine

☐ A is a sulphonamide
☐ B acts systemically to reduce inflammation
☐ C causes interstitial nephritis
☐ D leads to erythema multiforme
☐ E may cause gastrointestinal (GI) disturbance

2.15 A clinical trial should

☐ A be approved by the local ethics committee
☐ B specify the risks and benefits to the patient
☐ C include at least 100 subjects
☐ D include a 'control' group who receive no treatment
☐ E be randomised to avoid bias

2.16 Heparin

☐ A effects are reversed by vitamin K
☐ B can cause osteoporosis
☐ C acts by activating antithrombin III
☐ D takes 5 minutes to have effect when given orally
☐ E is monitored by measuring activated partial thromboplastin time (APTT)

2.17 Drugs that increase the effects of warfarin include

☐ A Rifampicin
☐ B Aspirin
☐ C Cimetidine
☐ D Cefuroxime
☐ E Chloral hydrate

2.18 Which of the following drugs are NOT used in parkinsonism?

☐ A Selegiline
☐ B Chlorpromazine
☐ C Methyldopa
☐ D Bromocriptine
☐ E Amantadine

2.19 The following drugs cause increased blood sugar:

- ☐ A Prednisolone
- ☐ B Furosemide (frusemide)
- ☐ C Propranolol
- ☐ D Glucagon
- ☐ E Methyldopa

2.20 A drug has a half-life of 18 hours. The following statements are true:

- ☐ A this means that the time taken for the plasma concentration to drop by 50% is 18 hours (following IV injection)
- ☐ B the drug must have a large volume of distribution
- ☐ C steady state concentration is achieved after three plasma half-lives ($t_{1/2}$)
- ☐ D a loading dose is likely to be required
- ☐ E it is eliminated by the liver

2.21 Gastrointestinal ulceration is caused by:

- ☐ A Potassium chloride
- ☐ B Diclofenac
- ☐ C Enteric-coated aspirin
- ☐ D Morphine
- ☐ E Paracetamol

2.22 Amiodarone

- ☐ A is used to treat ventricular fibrillation (VF)
- ☐ B causes slate-grey skin discoloration
- ☐ C has a half-life of 24 hours
- ☐ D prolongs the QT interval
- ☐ E enhances the effects of digoxin

2.23 Recognised treatments for diarrhoea include

- [ ] A   Codeine phosphate
- [ ] B   Misoprostol
- [ ] C   Lactulose
- [ ] D   Methylcellulose
- [ ] E   Senna

2.24 The following measures are used to lower blood pressure (BP):

- [ ] A   stopping smoking
- [ ] B   aerobic exercise
- [ ] C   decreasing alcohol intake
- [ ] D   increasing sodium intake
- [ ] E   reducing cholesterol

2.25 Hormone replacement therapy (HRT)

- [ ] A   reduces the risk of osteoporosis
- [ ] B   reduces the risk of breast cancer
- [ ] C   reduces cardiac disease
- [ ] D   should consist of progestogen if the uterus is intact
- [ ] E   causes vaginal atrophy

2.26 Isoniazid

- [ ] A   is antagonised by rifampicin
- [ ] B   causes hepatotoxicity
- [ ] C   may cause peripheral neuropathy which can be prevented by pyridoxine
- [ ] D   causes colour blindness
- [ ] E   is an enzyme inducer

2.27 The following statements are true:

☐   A   morphine should be given for nausea in patients with terminal disease

☐   B   buprenorphine may cause withdrawal symptoms in patients taking morphine

☐   C   morphine overdose should be treated with the antidote naltrexone

☐   D   NSAIDs are beneficial in osteoporosis

☐   E   morphine is appropriate for pain in a sickle cell crisis

2.28 The following statements are true:

☐   A   The plasma half life of a drug is the time taken to eliminate half the dose

☐   B   Steady state concentration is achieved after 3 to 5 half lives

☐   C   First pass metabolism is the concentration of drug excreted in the first hour

☐   D   Bioavailability is the amount of drug bound to receptors

☐   E   Absorption after intra-muscular injection is dependent on blood flow

2.29 Phaeochromocytoma

☐   A   causes hot flushes

☐   B   causes postural hypotension

☐   C   can be treated by laparoscopic adrenalectomy

☐   D   can be treated with phenoxybenzamine

☐   E   causes constipation

2.30 In hyperthyroidism

☐   A   radioactive iodine may be used as an appropriate treatment

☐   B   a goitre is always present

☐   C   a β-blocker such as propranolol may be used

☐   D   carbimazole may cause a goitre

☐   E   iodine is given orally

2.31 The following drugs cause cholestatic jaundice:

☐ A Alcohol
☐ B Chlorpromazine
☐ C Chlorpropamide
☐ D Halothane
☐ E Amoxicillin

2.32 The combined oral contraceptive pill

☐ A increases the risk of breast cancer
☐ B should be avoided if there is a history of deep vein thrombosis (DVT)
☐ C should be stopped if major surgery is planned within 4 weeks
☐ D contains oestrogen and progestogen
☐ E is used for hormone replacement therapy

2.33 The following are appropriate therapy in acute migraine:

☐ A Paracetamol and metoclopramide
☐ B Pizotifen
☐ C Ibuprofen
☐ D Propranolol
☐ E Sumatriptan

2.34 Lithium

☐ A is given intravenously to treat acute mania
☐ B toxicity may be precipitated by thiazide diuretics
☐ C should be stopped immediately after improvement of manic symptoms
☐ D is a monoamine-oxidase inhibitor
☐ E may cause hypothyroidism

2.35 The following are appropriate in the treatment of acute angle-closure glaucoma:

- ☐ A Mannitol
- ☐ B Adrenaline (epinephrine)
- ☐ C Acetazolamide
- ☐ D Atropine
- ☐ E Betaxolol

2.36 Aciclovir

- ☐ A is used to treat shingles
- ☐ B is a pro-drug
- ☐ C is the drug of choice for cytomegalovirus
- ☐ D is a guanosine derivative that inhibits viral DNA polymerase
- ☐ E is used for HIV infection

2.37 β_2-agonists

- ☐ A can be combined with corticosteroids to treat chronic asthma
- ☐ B cause bronchodilatation
- ☐ C increase intracellular cAMP
- ☐ D include dobutamine
- ☐ E include salmeterol
- ☐ F cause tremor

2.38 The following drugs should be stopped before a general anaesthetic for major surgery:

- ☐ A Lithium
- ☐ B Thyroxine
- ☐ C Combined oral contraceptive pill
- ☐ D Corticosteroids
- ☐ E Monoamine-oxidase inhibitors (MOAIs)

2.39 Treatment with high-dose oxygen is appropriate for a patient with:

- ☐ A   an acute asthmatic attack and a P_{CO_2} of 2.5 kPa
- ☐ B   an acute asthmatic attack and a P_{CO_2} of 6 kPa
- ☐ C   chronic obstructive pulmonary disease (COPD)
- ☐ D   pneumonia
- ☐ E   fibrosing alveolitis

2.40 Topical corticosteroids may be useful for the treatment of

- ☐ A   rosacea
- ☐ B   acne vulgaris
- ☐ C   urticaria
- ☐ D   eczema
- ☐ E   seborrhoeic dermatitis

2.41 The following concern diabetic patients on insulin:

- ☐ A   drivers need to inform the DVLA of their condition
- ☐ B   human insulin is always the preferred type
- ☐ C   insulin can be administered orally if injections are not tolerated
- ☐ D   insulin requirements increase during stress
- ☐ E   insulin should not be given if a patient is too ill to eat

2.42 Drugs which are effective in the prevention of motion sickness include

- ☐ A   Hyoscine
- ☐ B   Promethazine
- ☐ C   Cyclizine
- ☐ D   Metoclopramide
- ☐ E   Cinnarizine

2.43 Regarding vitamin/mineral supplements

☐   A   vitamin A should be given to all pregnant women
☐   B   folic acid should be taken in the last trimester of pregnancy
☐   C   fluoride confers significant resistance to dental caries
☐   D   all Asians should be given vitamin D supplements
☐   E   vitamin C reduces the duration of a cold

2.44 Clopidogrel

☐   A   causes thrombocytosis
☐   B   is a suitable substitute for aspirin in patients with peptic ulcer disease
☐   C   is contraindicated in patients with an acute coronary syndrome
☐   D   increases the risk of bleeding
☐   E   should not be given to patients already taking aspirin

2.45 Yellow card reporting

☐   A   should be used to report suspected reactions to drugs that have been on the market since 1982
☐   B   is used to report serious or unusual suspected reactions for all drugs
☐   C   is appropriate for minor suspected reactions for all drugs
☐   D   is used to report suspected reactions to vaccines
☐   E   cards can be completed by doctors, dentists and nurses

2.46 Oesophageal reflux may be treated with

☐   A   Metoclopramide
☐   B   Atropine sulphate
☐   C   Lansoprazole
☐   D   Ranitidine
☐   E   Loperamide

2.47 Prescriptions for controlled drugs (CDs)

☐ A   must be handwritten
☐ B   must be signed and dated by the doctor
☐ C   must contain the total amount of drugs in words and figures
☐ D   may not contain other drugs on the form
☐ E   may be given for 2 weeks' supply of drug to addicts in instalments

2.48 The following drugs are appropriate treatments for the paired neurological disorder:

☐ A   Tetrabenazine – Huntington's chorea
☐ B   Chlorpromazine – hiccup
☐ C   Propranolol – essential tremor
☐ D   Riluzole – motor neurone disease
☐ E   Botulinum toxin – blepharospasm

2.49 Sildenafil should not be prescribed to patients

☐ A   under 40 years of age
☐ B   over 70 years of age
☐ C   taking nitrate treatment
☐ D   with Parkinson's disease
☐ E   with diabetes

2.50 β-blockers are absolutely contraindicated in a patient with

☐ A   diabetes
☐ B   asthma
☐ C   heart failure
☐ D   mild peripheral vascular disease
☐ E   Alzheimer's disease

PAPER 2

Answers

The correct answer options for each question are given below.

2.1	A B	2.26	B C
2.2	B D	2.27	B E
2.3	B D	2.28	B E
2.4	A B D	2.29	A C D E
2.5	B C	2.30	A D E
2.6	C D E	2.31	B C
2.7	B D E	2.32	A B C D
2.8	B D E	2.33	A C E
2.9	B D E	2.34	B E
2.10	A B C E	2.35	A C E
2.11	A B C	2.36	A D
2.12	A C D	2.37	A B C E
2.13	A B	2.38	A C E
2.14	C E	2.39	A B D E
2.15	A B E	2.40	D E
2.16	B C E	2.41	A D
2.17	B C D E	2.42	A B C E
2.18	B C	2.43	C
2.19	A D	2.44	B D
2.20	A C D	2.45	B D E
2.21	A B C	2.46	A C D
2.22	A B D E	2.47	A B C E
2.23	A D	2.48	A B C D E
2.24	B C	2.49	C
2.25	A C D	2.50	B

MCQs
Paper 2
Answers and teaching notes

2.1 Thrombolysis   Answers: A B

The major contraindications to thrombolytic therapy are:

- aortic dissection
- active bleeding
- stroke within 1 year
- major surgery in the last 2 months
- acute pericarditis
- haemophilia
- pregnancy

The relative contraindications are:

- anticoagulant therapy
- high blood pressure, > 200/110
- previous stroke with deficit
- active peptic ulcer disease
- organ biopsy in the previous 2 weeks
- cavitating pulmonary disease
- minor surgery within the last month

2.2 Side-effects   Answers: B D

Thiazide diuretics promote sodium and water excretion; the main side-effects include hypokalaemia, hyponatraemia, metabolic alkalosis, increased plasma uric acid, hypovolaemia, postural hypotension, hyperglycaemia, increased triglyceride concentrations, and impotence. Furosemide (frusemide) is a loop or 'high ceiling' diuretic that causes sodium and water excretion, and adverse effects are hypokalaemia, hypovolaemia and metabolic alkalosis. Amiodarone is an effective antiarrhythmic but has many side-effects, which include photosensitivity, slate-grey skin discoloration, thyroid dysfunction, pulmonary fibrosis and corneal deposits. Bromocriptine is a dopamine agonist and is used to treat hyperprolactinaemia, galactorrhoea and Parkinson's disease. Unwanted effects are dizziness, constipation, postural hypotension, nausea and vomiting. NSAIDs are very commonly used drugs, their actions are: anti-inflammatory, analgesic and antipyretic. Side-effects are gastrointestinal disturbance, including nausea, vomiting, diarrhoea, dyspepsia, peptic ulceration, skin rashes, **renal toxicity**, bone marrow disturbance, liver impairment and bronchospasm which may precipitate asthma in susceptible patients.

2.3 Pituitary ablation   Answers: B D

The pituitary gland is divided into anterior and posterior components. The anterior pituitary secretes: adrenocorticotrophic hormone (ACTH), growth hormone (GH), gonadotrophins – follicle stimulating hormone (FSH) and luteinising hormone (LH), thyroid stimulating hormone (TSH), prolactin and melanocyte stimulating hormone. The posterior pituitary gland consists of nerve cells that release peptides, namely oxytocin and vasopressin (antidiuretic hormone). Insulin is produced by the pancreas. The loss of ACTH can precipitate an Addisonian crisis and glucocorticoids must be replaced. Fludrocortisone is a substitute mineralocorticoid, like aldosterone, which is not affected.

2.4 Myocardial infarction   Answers: A B D

Coronary vessel thrombosis results in infarction of a segment of myocardium. This may result in ventricular failure or dysrhythmias, and hence mortality. Prevention of irreversible ischaemic damage of cardiac cells is therefore important, and forms the basis of numerous studies. β-blockers reduce cardiac work. They have a small benefit when given immediately for acute MI as shown in the ISIS-1 (International Study of Infarct Survival). They also show benefit in long-term use. Angiotensin-converting enzyme inhibitors improve survival when given soon after an MI as shown in clinical trials. Nitrates reduce cardiac work but, in the ISIS-4 trial, did not influence the clinical outcome after myocardial infarction. The benefit of aspirin was shown in ISIS-2. Furosemide (frusemide) gives effective symptomatic relief from pulmonary oedema, and is often required after MI, but does not influence survival.

2.5 *Clostridium difficile* Answers: B C

Treatment with broad-spectrum antibiotics, e.g. cephalosporins or clindamycin may result in 'pseudomembranous colitis' due to overgrowth of *Clostridium difficile.* Vancomycin is poorly absorbed and is given orally to eradicate *C. difficile* from the gut. Metronidazole is also effective. The patient must be rehydrated with IV fluids to replace volume loss that occurs secondary to diarrhoea. Omeprazole is a proton pump inhibitor, and is used to decrease gastric acid production.

2.6 Digoxin Answers: C D E

Digoxin slows ventricular rate in atrial fibrillation. Elimination is mainly by renal excretion, and care must be taken in the elderly and in patients with renal failure. Adverse effects include nausea, vomiting, cardiac arrhythmias and confusion. Digoxin has a narrow therapeutic index, and toxicity can be precipitated by drugs that reduce renal clearance, e.g. verapamil or amiodarone. Loop diuretics reduce plasma potassium, increasing the effect of digoxin. Both drugs are often given simultaneously, and K^+ requires close monitoring.

2.7 Therapeutic drug monitoring Answers: B D E

TDM is necessary for those drugs that have a narrow therapeutic index, i.e. a narrow concentration range in which a drug is effective and above which the drug has toxic effects, and where there is a close relationship between plasma concentration and the risk of adverse events.

$$\text{The therapeutic index} = \frac{\text{maximum non-toxic dose}}{\text{minimum effective dose}}$$
$$\text{(ratio)}$$

Serious dose-related toxic effects can be avoided by either reducing the dosage or increasing the length of time between doses. Other examples include gentamicin, and vancomycin. Warfarin concentrations are not checked; the prothrombin time (INR) is used for pharmacodynamic monitoring.

2.8 Metronidazole   Answers: B D E

Metronidazole can be used orally, intravenously, rectally, vaginally, or topically. It is active against anaerobic bacteria and protozoa, including trichomonal infection, *Gardnerella vaginalis*, *Entamoeba histolytica*, and *Giardia lamblia*. It is often used for prophylaxis in surgery, especially where there is a risk of exposure to colonic anaerobic bacteria. Side-effects are nausea and vomiting, rashes, leucopenia, gastrointestinal disturbance, hepatitis and peripheral neuropathy, and it interacts with alcohol leading to accumulation of acetaldehyde which can cause vomiting, arrhythmias and hypotension. Metronidazole must be given orally to treat pseudomembranous colitis, as an alternative to vancomycin treatment.

2.9 Suxamethonium   Answers: B D E

Suxamethonium is a depolarising muscle relaxant with a rapid onset of action and short duration of action. It mimics acetylcholine at the neuromuscular junction. Its action cannot be reversed and therefore paralysis occurs until spontaneous recovery. Anticholinesterases such as neostigmine potentiate neuromuscular block. Prolonged paralysis may occur in patients with low or atypical plasma cholinesterase. Suxamethonium usually causes painful muscle fasciculation prior to paralysis, and this effect may be seen after surgery. Atropine is given for bradycardia or excess salivation associated with repeated doses of suxamethonium.

2.10 Nephrotoxic drugs   Answers: A B C E

A number of different drugs characteristically cause impaired renal

function. Gentamicin is nephrotoxic and ototoxic; b(
dependent adverse effects; therapeutic drug monitoring
useful, and aminoglycosides should be used with cautio(___ents
with renal impairment and reduced drug clearance. NSAIDs, including diclofenac, can cause acute tubular necrosis, or papillary necrosis (particularly in combination with paracetamol). Ciclosporin is
nephrotoxic, and cleared predominantly by the kidneys. Therefore,
as ciclosporin concentrations rise, renal function deteriorates further; therapeutic drug monitoring is used to reduce the risk of renal
damage. Furosemide (frusemide) causes diuresis but can also cause
renal failure. NSAIDs are nephrotoxic, particularly in high dose, and
should be used with care in patients with impaired renal blood flow.
Amoxicillin is not directly nephrotoxic.

2.11 Lidocaine (lignocaine)   Answers: A B C

Lidocaine (lignocaine) is administered intravenously for ventricular
arrhythmias. It can cause ventricular fibrillation in toxic doses. It is
also rapidly absorbed from the oral mucosa. Lidocaine (lignocaine)
blocks Na^+ channels and exerts its anaesthetic effect by inhibiting
nerve conduction. Its greatest effects are on small nerve fibres,
reducing pain and temperature sensation before reducing conduction in proprioception and motor fibres. It is metabolised by liver
enzymes.

2.12 Morphine   Answers: A C D

Opioids are agonists at central opiate receptors, and reduce the
perception of pain. This reduces distress and sympathetic outflow,
which is of benefit in myocardial infarction or acute left ventricular
failure. Furthermore, they reduce respiratory 'sensation' and suppress the cough reflex and sensation of pulmonary oedema. They do
however cause hypotension, cardiorespiratory depression, and constipation. Morphine can be administered by subcutaneous infusion
as the basis of patient-controlled analgesia, although diamorphine is
often preferred because smaller quantities need to be infused to
obtain the same effect. Morphine and diamorphine are thought to
promote biliary spasm, and pethidine is often the preferred analgesic
choice for biliary colic. Opiates often **cause** nausea and, paradoxically, they can cause headache. For this reason, they are often

administered with an anti-emetic.

2.13 Status epilepticus   Answers: A B

Status epilepticus is treated with IV lorazepam or diazepam. However, rectal diazepam solutions can be used, if this allows more rapid administration. Establishing an airway and administering oxygen 60% is important, although higher concentrations may be required. Slow IV phenytoin is given to prevent recurrence. The absorption of intramuscular phenytoin is too unpredictable, and usually slower. Clomethiazole is given in resistant cases, as is paraldehyde. Flumazenil is a diazepam antidote.

2.14 Mesalazine   Answers: C E

Mesalazine is 5-acetylsalicylic acid (5-ASA), and sulfasalazine is a combination of sulphapyridine and 5-ASA. 5-ASA is the active moiety, which is released in the colon when the bacterial flora cleaves the sulphonamide component. Mesalazine may cause gastrointestinal upset, diarrhoea, and interstitial nephritis. Sulphonamides cause GI disturbance, low sperm count and erythema multiforme.

2.15 Clinical trials   Answers: A B E

Clinical trials may be designed to compare a new 'test' drug with an existing 'standard' drug or with no drug at all, in which case a 'placebo' drug is administered. The use of a control group is essential to validate the results. However, the control group can receive a matching placebo or active comparator drug. Randomisation and 'blinding' both help to avoid bias. Patients must give 'informed' consent to participate, and a local research ethics committee must have approved the protocol. The number of subjects to be included in the study is calculated statistically and varies depending on the outcome variable and likely magnitude of the expected effect.

2.16 Heparin   Answers: B C E

Effects of heparin are reversed by protamine sulphate, whereas warfarin is reversed by vitamin K. Chronic use results in osteoporosis and alopecia. Heparin activates antithrombin III, which inactivates factor X and thrombin. Heparin acts immediately following IV administration. It is not absorbed from the gut, and hence not active if administered orally. Dose is adjusted according to APTT, whereas warfarin is adjusted by prothrombin time (PT) or INR.

2.17 Warfarin   Answers: B C D E

Rifampicin induces liver enzymes, which metabolise warfarin more rapidly and reduce its effects. Other inducers are barbiturates, carbamazepine and griseofulvin. Aspirin and NSAIDs increase the risk of bleeding in combination with warfarin. Drugs that inhibit hepatic metabolism, and potentiate its effects, include cimetidine, imipramine, metronidazole, amiodarone, and ciprofloxacin. Cefuroxime acts as an enzyme inhibitor. Chloral hydrate displaces warfarin from albumin binding sites and increases the 'free', active portion.

2.18 Parkinsonism   Answers: B C

Selegiline is a monoamine-oxidase-B inhibitor that prevents dopamine (DA) breakdown. Chlorpromazine is an antipsychotic with dopamine antagonist properties, that can cause parkinsonism. It is levodopa, is the precursor of DA; methyldopa is an antihypertensive. Bromocriptine causes direct stimulation of DA receptors, and amantadine stimulates release of DA from central neurones.

2.19 Blood sugar   Answers: A D

Glucocorticoids stimulate glycogenolysis. Thiazides, but not loop diuretics, raise blood sugar. Propranolol is a β-blocker, which causes modest increases in LDL cholesterol, but does not increase blood glucose. Glucagon can be given as emergency treatment for hypoglycaemia, as it mobilises hepatic glycogen stores. Methyldopa can cause pancreatitis, but does not directly influence blood sugar.

2.20 Half-life   Answers: A C D

By definition, plasma $t_{1/2}$ depends on volume of distribution and clearance; therefore, volume of distribution is not necessarily large. Steady state concentration is achieved after approximately 3–5 half-lives, regardless of the half-life itself. In this case, steady state concentrations may not be achieved for several days, and a loading dose will be required. Half-life does not give any indication of the route of drug clearance.

2.21 Gastrointestinal ulceration   Answers: A B C

Potassium chloride causes gastrointestinal ulceration, in the stomach or small bowel. NSAIDs and aspirin can cause peptic ulceration, and gastrointestinal blood loss from the stomach, small bowel, and (in a small number of cases) the large bowel. Enteric coating of aspirin only reduces its irritant effect. Morphine and paracetamol do not cause ulceration of the gastrointestinal tract and, therefore, are safe in patients with peptic ulcer disease.

2.22 Amiodarone   Answers: A B D E

Amiodarone is used to treat: supraventricular tachycardia, ventricular tachycardia, atrial fibrillation/atrial flutter, ventricular fibrillation. Slate-grey skin discoloration is one of many side-effects. Others are corneal deposits, peripheral neuropathy, hypothyroidism and hyperthyroidism, pulmonary fibrosis, jaundice/hepatitis, metallic taste, impotence, alopecia and benign raised intracranial pressure. It has a very long half-life of 4–6 weeks. Digoxin plasma concentration increases due to reduced clearance. Amiodarone does prolong the QT interval.

2.23 Diarrhoea   Answers: A D

Treatments for diarrhoea:	*Causes of diarrhoea – laxatives:*
Rehydration	Bulking agents (methylcellulose, ispaghula)
Adsorbents and bulking agent kaolin,methylcellulose, for diarrhoea associated with diverticular disease	Stimulants, e.g. senna, ispaghula, bisacodyl, dantron, Docusol®, sodium picosulfate

Antimotility drugs e.g. codeine/opiates, loperamide	Osmotic laxatives – lactulose Faecal softeners, e.g. arachis oil

Opiates can be used for symptomatic relief. Misoprostol causes diarrhoea, and lactulose is used to treat constipation. Methylcellulose is used to cause bulking of stool and can treat diarrhoea or constipation. Senna is a stimulant laxative.

2.24 Lowering blood pressure   Answers: B C

Hypertension and smoking are not associated but both are important risk factors for ischaemic heart disease. 40 minutes of exercise, four times per week, is expected to reduce BP by 5 mmHg. Chronic high intake of alcohol raises BP. Increasing Na^+ intake causes increased fluid retention and raised BP. Reduction of cholesterol reduces ischaemic heart disease risk.

2.25 HRT   Answers: A C D

HRT reduces the risk of osteoporosis and fractures in the elderly. The effects on breast cancer risk are not adequately proven, although there may be a modest increased risk. Oestrogens are protective of the heart in women, and HRT reduces the incidence of strokes and myocardial infarction. Oestrogens increase the risk of endometrial cancer and this is opposed by progestogens. Vaginal oestrogens are used topically to treat atrophy.

2.26 Isoniazid   Answers: B C

Isoniazid and rifampicin are given in combination for the treatment of TB. Hepatic function should be monitored regularly. Peripheral neuropathy is a common side-effect. Ethambutol causes visual disturbances, including loss of accuracy and colour blindness. Ethambutol can interfere with retinal function, and stopping the drug usually reverses the visual side-effects. Rifampicin is an enzyme inducer.

2.27 Morphine   Answers: B E

Morphine causes nausea. It should be given with an anti-emetic. Buprenorphine has both agonist and antagonist actions. The antagonistic actions may precipitate withdrawal. In morphine overdose naloxone is the antidote. Naltrexone is an opioid antagonist used for opioid dependence to prevent the euphoria effect. NSAIDs are used for osteoarthritis (OA). Severe pain occurs in sickle cell; there is a risk of tolerance and dependence.

2.28 Correct statements   Answers: B E

The plasma half life (t1/2) is the time taken for the plasma concentration of the drug to fall to half its value from any starting point. The plasma concentration is not the dose given. Steady state concentration is generally achieved after about 3 half lives. This can be achieved sooner if a larger 'loading' dose is given as seen with digoxin. First pass metabolism is the amount of drug that is metabolised by the liver after absorption from the gut, via the portal venous system. Examples of drugs that undergo considerable 1st pass elimination are aspirin, chlorpromazine, pethidine, morphine, propranolol, glyceryl trinitrate and salbutamol. Other routes of administration such as sublingual, avoids the 1st pass effect. Bioavailability is the amount of drug in the systemic circulation and available at the site of action. It takes into account both absorption and local degradation. Intra-muscular injection produces a faster effect than oral administration. Absorption is increased by increasing local blood flow and reduced in circulatory failure. Absorption also depends on diffusion through the tissue.

2.29 Phaeochromocytoma   Answers: A C D E

Phaeochromocytoma is a catecholamine-secreting tumour producing sympathetic stimulation. Clinical features of phaeochromocytoma are severe hypertension, sweating, hot flushes, and pallor. The effects can be episodic. Surgical removal of the adrenal gland tumour is the treatment of choice. Phenoxybenzamine and phentolamine (short-acting) are used for α-blockade and, after α-blockade, β-blockers can be used for extra blood pressure lowering effects and to treat tachycardia.

2.30 Hyperthyroidism   Answers: A D E

Radioactive iodine is given orally. It is taken up by the thyroid gland and emits β radiation which affects the thyroid cells. Hyperthyroidism may be due to Graves' disease in which case a goitre may not be present. A β blocker, e.g. propranolol is used for tachycardia. Thyroxine production is blocked by carbimazole and the resulting loss of negative feedback causes increased TSH release. This may cause a goitre. A small dose of thyroxine can be given with carbimazole to avoid this. Iodine transiently ↓ thyroid hormone secretion and reduces the vascularity of the gland. This is helpful if surgery is planned.

2.31 Cholestatic jaundice   Answers: B C

Drug-induced cholestatic jaundice is due to intrahepatic biliary obstruction. Drugs may cause hepatocellular damage or cholestatic jaundice. It is worth knowing a basic list for each of these:

Hepatotoxicity is caused by:	Cholestatic jaundice is caused by:
Paracetamol	Methyltestosterone
Aspirin	Chlorpropamide
Alcohol	Tolbutamide
MAOIs	Chlorpromazine
Halothane	Erythromycin estolate
Phenytoin	

In hepatic failure, drugs which are metabolised by hepatic enzymes accumulate and their effects are enhanced or prolonged. Alcohol causes liver cirrhosis. 17α-substituted testosterone causes cholestatic jaundice. Erythromycin estolate, in particular, is known to do this. Other forms do not have the same effect.

2.32 The combined oral contraceptive pill   Answers: A B C D

The risk of breast cancer is associated with exposure to oestrogen. The oral contraceptive pill should be avoided in patients with a history of previous breast cancer. There is an increased risk of venous thrombosis in pregnancy, as well as while taking the oral contraceptive pill.

Incidence of thromboembolism:

- in non-pregnant women = 5/100,000/year
- on oral contraceptive pill = 15/100,000/year
- in pregnancy = 60/100,000/year

The risk factors for venous thromboembolic disease are:

- positive family history
- obesity
- immobilisation
- varicose veins

Oestrogen-containing contraception is not advised. Progestogen-only preparations may be used. HRT consists of a different dosage of oestrogen and progestogen from the oral contraceptive pill. Whilst on HRT, a woman may still be fertile.

2.33 Acute migraine   Answers: A C E

The treatment of migraine should be considered in two phases – the acute attack and prophylaxis of migraine. Acute attacks respond to analgesics such as aspirin, paracetamol, NSAIDs, to specific $5HT_1$ agonists such as sumatriptan, or ergotamine. For nausea, an anti-emetic is added. Metoclopramide and domperidone are suitable anti-emetics and have the added advantage of increasing gastric emptying. Prophylaxis of migraine consists of:

- avoidance of precipitating factors, e.g. cheese, chocolate
- pizotifen = antihistamine and 5HT antagonist
- β-blockers, e.g. propranolol
- tricyclic antidepressants, e.g. amitriptyline
- sodium valproate (but not phenytoin)
- cyproheptadine/nifedipine are occasionally used

2.34 Lithium   Answers: B E

Lithium salts are used to treat and prevent mania in bipolar affective disorder, and to treat unipolar depression. It is given orally in tablet form. Lithium has a narrow therapeutic index, effective at a range of

0.4–1 mmol/l. Toxicity becomes more likely above this, and especially beyond 1.5 mmol/l, and plasma levels should be monitored regularly. The toxic effects include nausea, vomiting, diarrhoea, ataxia, tremor, dysarthria, nystagmus, renal failure and convulsions. Long-term use may cause hypothyroidism and goitre. Toxicity is precipitated by sodium depletion – so care must be taken with concurrent use of thiazide diuretics. Abrupt withdrawal of lithium can result in a relapse of symptoms and it therefore should be withdrawn gradually. Lithium has a long half-life, of approximately 12 hours.

2.35 Acute angle-closure glaucoma   Answers: A C E

Raised intraocular pressure (IOP) is associated with glaucoma and can cause blindness. There is continued secretion of aqueous humour into the anterior chamber but drainage out is impeded by dilation of the pupil. Muscarinic agonists constrict the pupil and lower IOP. Treatment – in emergency includes mannitol 20% IV infusion or acetazolamide IV to lower IOP. Drugs that lower IOP are:

- Pilocarpine – muscarinic agonist – eye drops
- Betaxolol, timolol – β-blockers – eye drops
- Acetazolamide – carbonic anhydrase inhibitor – systemic
- Apraclonidine – α_2-adrenoceptor agonist – eye drops
- Carbachol – eye drops

Surgery – iridectomy, drainage of aqueous humour. Adrenaline reduces the rate of production of aqueous humour and increases outflow. It does however cause pupil dilation (mydriasis) and is therefore contraindicated in the acute attack. Atropine is a muscarinic antagonist and can be dangerous in angle-closure glaucoma.

2.36 Aciclovir   Answers: A D

Aciclovir is used to treat:

- Varicella-zoster infection – shingles: oral for immunocompetent patients; IV for immunocompromised patients
- Herpes simplex infection – genital, mucocutaneous, conjunctivitis, encephalitis

• Varicella – chickenpox, in immunocompromised patients

It reaches high concentrations in cerebrospinal fluid (CSF). It is excreted by the kidney. Valaciclovir is a pro-drug of aciclovir. It is converted to the monophosphate and then to triphosphate which inhibits viral DNA polymerase. It is more potent against the herpes virus enzyme than host enzyme. Ganciclovir is the treatment of choice for cytomegalovirus. Zidovudine and abacavir are used for HIV infection. Aciclovir has a role in the immunocompromised patient as prophylaxis or treatment of herpes infection.

2.37 β_2-agonists: Answers: A B C E

Stimulation of β_2-receptors causes relaxation of smooth muscle. Activation of adenylate cyclase causes a rise in intracellular cAMP. This activates a protein kinase which phosphorylates myosin kinase and inhibits contraction. Selective β_2 agonists are used to treat asthma: salbutamol and terbutaline are short acting (~3 hours) and can be given by aerosol inhalation, orally or iv; salmeterol is long-acting, given by aerosol inhalation (~12 hours). Inhaled steroids can be used regularly to prevent acute attacks. In acute exacerbation, a short course of oral prednisolone is advised. Dobutamine is a selective β_1 agonist which ↑ cardiac contractility. Side-effects of β_2 agonists are: fine tremor, headache, palpitations, arrhythmias, peripheral vasodilatation.

2.38 Drugs to be stopped before major surgery   Answers: A C E

Lithium should be stopped 24 hours before major surgery but can be continued for minor surgery if there is careful monitoring of fluids and electrolytes.

The combined oral contraceptive pill should be stopped because of its thromboembolic effects. MAOIs have potentially hazardous interactions and should normally be stopped 2 weeks before surgery.

Antiepileptics, antipsychotics, bronchodilators, cardiovascular drugs and thyroid or antithyroid drugs should not normally be stopped before surgery.

If a patient is or has been taking steroids, then corticosteroid cover must be given during the anaesthetic and the immediate post-operative period.

2.39 Treatment with high-dose oxygen   Answers: A B D E

In conditions where hypoventilation is likely, e.g. COPD, high-dose oxygen must not be given. This is because some patients who retain CO_2 rely on a low PO_2 to produce a hypoxic drive for ventilation. If high concentration oxygen is given the drive for ventilation is stopped and the patient may cease breathing.

High-dose oxygen (i.e. up to a concentration of 60%) is appropriate when conditions produce hyperventilation, such as an acute asthma attack, pneumonia, pulmonary embolism and fibrosing alveolitis. In these conditions a low PO_2 is associated with a normal or low PCO_2.

An important exception is in a life-threatening attack of asthma. The patient may become so exhausted that hypoventilation results, causing a decrease in arterial oxygen tension and a rise in PCO_2. In this case a high concentration of oxygen is required and positive-pressure ventilation should be urgently considered.

2.40 Topical corticosteroids   Answers: D E

Topical corticosteroids are used in the treatment of eczema, seborrhoeic dermatitis and psoriasis. Topical corticosteroids are of no value in the treatment of urticaria. They are contraindicated in rosacea. Corticosteroids predispose to the development of acne vulgaris.

2.41 Insulin   Answers: A D

Drivers treated with insulin or oral antidiabetic drugs are required to notify the DVLA of their condition. (Drivers of heavy goods vehicles or public service vehicles whose diabetes is controlled by diet alone must also notify the DVLA.)

Insulin may be extracted from pork or beef pancreas, but beef insulins are now rarely used. Human sequence insulin may be produced by enzymatic modification of porcine insulin or biosynthetically by recombinant DNA technology. All insulin preparations are immunogenic in man, although this rarely causes a problem in clinical practice.

No real advantage of human insulin has been shown in clinical trials. Some patients have found that switching to human insulin from porcine insulin has been associated with a reduction in warning symptoms of hypoglycaemia. Insulin is inactivated by gastrointestinal enzymes and must be given by injection.

Insulin requirements often increase during illness, stress, trauma, puberty and during the second and third trimesters of pregnancy. Requirements may be decreased in renal and hepatic impairment and in some endocrine disorders, e.g. Addison's disease and hypopituitarism.

Blood glucose levels rise if insulin is not given and during illness it rises further due to the effect of stress hormones, e.g. cortisol. During an illness a patient is particularly at risk of hyperglycaemia and insulin is absolutely necessary. In fact, higher doses may be needed.

2.42 Motion sickness   Answers: A B C E

The most effective drug for prevention of motion sickness is hyoscine. Antihistamines are less effective but are better tolerated as they have fewer side-effects. If a sedative effect is required promethazine is useful, but generally a less sedating antihistamine such as cyclizine, or cinnarizine, is preferred. Metoclopramide acts selectively on the chemoreceptor trigger zone in the brain and is ineffective in motion sickness.

2.43 Vitamin/mineral supplements   Answer: C

Evidence suggests that high levels of vitamin A may cause birth defects and women who are pregnant or about to become pregnant should not take vitamin A supplements (including fish-oil drops) except on the advice of a doctor.

Folic acid should be started as soon as a woman starts to try to conceive and should be continued for the first 12 weeks of pregnancy. Folic acid has been shown to reduce the incidence of neural tube defects.

Fluoride confers significant resistance to dental caries. The topical action of fluoride on enamel and dentine is more important than its systemic effect. Systemic fluoride supplements should not be prescribed without knowing how much fluoride is in the local water supply.

Vitamin C has not been proved to reduce the duration of a cold or improve symptoms.

2.44 Clopidogrel: Answers: B D

Clopidogrel is an antiplatelet drug used in both the treatment and prevention of acute coronary syndromes. The combination of clopidogrel and aspirin has been shown to be more effective than either alone in treatment of certain patients with acute coronary syndrome. As with aspirin, there is an increased risk of intracerebral haemorrhage.

Clopidogrel has fewer side-effects than aspirin and is a suitable substitute for aspirin in patients with peptic ulceration. Side-effects include neutropenia.

2.45 Yellow card reporting   Answers: B D E

Yellow cards should be used to report all suspected reactions (minor or severe) to new medicines including recently introduced vaccinations.

Yellow cards should also be used to report serious suspected reactions to established medicines – even if the reaction is well recognised already. Minor reactions of established drugs should not be reported with yellow cards.

Doctors, dentists, coroners, pharmacists and (more recently) nurses are allowed to complete a yellow card report.

2.46 Oesophageal reflux   Answers: A C D

Metoclopramide is a centrally acting dopamine antagonist. In addition, within the GI tract it releases acetylcholine which:

(a) increases motility and increases emptying
(b) produces oesophageal spasm that prevents reflux.

Atropine blocks these effects. Lansoprazole and ranitidine decrease acid production and therefore reduce acid reflux. Loperamide is an opiate agonist and is used to treat diarrhoea.

2.47 Prescriptions for controlled drugs   Answers: A B C E

Prescriptions for controlled drugs should:

1. be signed and dated by the doctor
2. specify the doctor's address
3. be in the prescriber's handwriting, with:
   • the name and address of the patient
   • the form and strength of preparation
   • the total quantity in both words and figures
   • the dose

In certain cases, the dispensing pharmacist can be instructed to dispense the prescription in instalments to help manage patients with drug addiction.

2.48 Treatments for neurological disorders   Answers: A B C D E

Tetrabenazine is mainly used to control movement disorders in Huntington's chorea and related disorders. Its use may be limited by the development of depression. Chlorpromazine and haloperidol are used to relieve intractable hiccups. Propranolol or other β-blockers may be useful in treating essential tremor, or tremor associated with anxiety and thyrotoxicosis. Riluzole extends the life and delays the need for mechanical ventilation in a proportion of patients with amyotrophic lateral sclerosis. Botulinum toxin can be used to paralyse muscles in the treatment of hemifacial spasm and torticollis.

2.49 Sildenafil   Answer: C

Sildenafil (Viagra) is used for the treatment of erectile dysfunction. It must not be given to patients receiving treatment with nitrates due to the risk of hypotension. It is also contraindicated in patients with recent stroke or myocardial infarction, blood pressure below 90/50 mmHg and hereditary degenerative retinal disorders. Side-effects include dyspepsia, headache, flushing, dizziness, visual disturbances and increased intraocular pressure. An important use of the drug is to treat erectile dysfunction in men who have an organic cause for this, e.g. diabetes, multiple sclerosis, Parkinson's disease, poliomyelitis or spina bifida.

2.50 β-blockers   Answer: B

The important part of the question is the word 'absolutely', which implies that the drug should never be given under any circumstance. The warning symptoms and signs of hypoglycaemia are reduced by β-blockers, and diabetes is a relative contraindication. While β-blockers can impair cardiac output, they are of benefit in selected patients with heart failure and appear to reduce mortality due to arrhythmias. Many patients with peripheral vascular disease can tolerate β-blockers, but if symptoms worsen, the drug should be withdrawn. β-blockers should not be prescribed in severe peripheral vascular disease. β-blockers (even in the form of eye drops) must not be given to patients with asthma; even cardioselective β-blockers can provoke asthma and make inhaled β-agonists ineffective.

Multiple Choice Questions

PAPER 3

Questions (answers, page 82)

50 questions: time allowed, 2 hours.
Mark your answers with a tick (True) or a cross (False) in the box provided. Leave the box blank for 'Don't know'. Do not look at the answers until you have completed the whole question paper.

3.1 The adverse effects of ACE inhibitors include

- ☐ A   taste disturbance
- ☐ B   persistent dry cough
- ☐ C   hypertension
- ☐ D   impotence
- ☐ E   diabetic nephropathy

3.2 Isoniazid

- ☐ A   is used in the treatment of tuberculosis
- ☐ B   may cause liver toxicity
- ☐ C   has unwanted effects that are enhanced by pyridoxine
- ☐ D   is excreted in the urine
- ☐ E   interacts with carbamazepine
- ☐ F   metabolism depends on acetylation

3.3 Captopril

☐ A is an angiotensin II antagonist
☐ B causes first-dose hypertension
☐ C may cause cough
☐ D does not lower BP in patients with renal artery stenosis
☐ E does not lower BP in patients with heart failure

3.4 The following are recognised treatments for acute left ventricular failure:

☐ A 100% oxygen
☐ B Dobutamine
☐ C Diamorphine
☐ D 200J DC shock
☐ E IV adrenaline (epinephrine)

3.5 Thiazide diuretics

☐ A cause hypercalcaemia
☐ B cause hyperglycaemia
☐ C may cause an acute attack of gout
☐ D reduce BP and the risk of stroke
☐ E cause hypercholesterolaemia

3.6 Carbimazole

☐ A is converted to a pro-drug
☐ B may cause cough
☐ C can be used in pregnancy
☐ D inhibits thyroxine production
☐ E inhibits the conversion T_4 to T_3

3.7 Sodium cromoglicate

- ☐ A is of no value in the treatment of an acute asthmatic attack
- ☐ B is of no value in exercise-induced asthma
- ☐ C is more effective in adults than children
- ☐ D may cause bronchospasm
- ☐ E should not be used for more than 1 week at a time

3.8 Leukotriene receptor antagonists

- ☐ A act by inhibiting prostaglandin action
- ☐ B are indicated in the treatment of an acute severe asthma attack
- ☐ C should not be prescribed concurrently with steroids
- ☐ D have no significant side-effects
- ☐ E are administered using an inhaler

3.9 Drugs that act on the central nervous system (CNS) include

- ☐ A Phenobarbitone
- ☐ B Domperidone
- ☐ C Levodopa
- ☐ D Benserazide
- ☐ E Carbidopa

3.10 Drugs for the treatment of Alzheimer's disease

- ☐ A should only be initiated by a specialist
- ☐ B should be stopped if improvement has not occurred within 1 week
- ☐ C should be given as weekly IM injections
- ☐ D are inhibitors of acetylcholinesterase
- ☐ E have a more marked effect if the disease is severe

3.11 Benzodiazepines have the following effects:

- ☐ A   sedation
- ☐ B   amnesia
- ☐ C   anxiolysis
- ☐ D   analgesia
- ☐ E   respiratory depression

3.12 The following may cause bleeding from the gastrointestinal tract:

- ☐ A   Indometacin
- ☐ B   Ferrous sulphate
- ☐ C   Atenolol
- ☐ D   Lansoprazole
- ☐ E   Aminophylline

3.13 The following drugs can precipitate or exacerbate asthma:

- ☐ A   Aspirin
- ☐ B   Prednisolone
- ☐ C   Paracetamol
- ☐ D   Codeine phosphate
- ☐ E   Diazepam

3.14 The following are true of analgesics:

- ☐ A   they are more effective in preventing than treating pain
- ☐ B   opioids are the first-line treatment for pain from bone metastases
- ☐ C   morphine cannot be given orally
- ☐ D   fentanyl can be given as a patch
- ☐ E   diamorphine can be given subcutaneously

3.15 Healing of a peptic ulcer can be promoted by

- ☐ A   bland diet
- ☐ B   chlorphenamine (chlorpheniramine)
- ☐ C   bismuth colloid
- ☐ D   ranitidine
- ☐ E   exercise

3.16 The following are true of lipid-lowering drugs:

☐ A the aim of treatment is to lower HDL and raise LDL cholesterol
☐ B they are only effective in secondary prevention of coronary heart disease
☐ C statins are used to treat hypercholesterolaemia
☐ D fibrates are used to treat hypertriglyceridaemia
☐ E rhabdomyolysis is a common complication

3.17 The following procedures should be covered by antibiotic prophylaxis in a patient with a prosthetic valve:

☐ A tonsillectomy
☐ B sigmoidoscopy
☐ C barium enema
☐ D removal of an intrauterine contraceptive device (IUCD)
☐ E bronchoscopy

3.18 The following are drugs of choice for the listed types of meningitis:

		Type of meningitis	Drugs
☐	A	pneumococcal	gentamicin
☐	B	meningococcal	amoxicillin
☐	C	*Haemophilus*	cefotaxime
☐	D	*Listeria*	ampicillin and gentamicin
☐	E	unknown organism	penicillin V

3.19 Trimethoprim is an appropriate treatment for the following genitourinary conditions:

☐ A cystitis
☐ B prostatitis
☐ C epididymo-orchitis
☐ D pyelonephritis
☐ E atrophic vaginitis

3.20 Gastric lavage is contraindicated in an overdose of

- ☐ A Iron
- ☐ B Caustic soda
- ☐ C Aspirin
- ☐ D Theophylline
- ☐ E Lithium

3.21 The following drugs cause constipation:

- ☐ A Loperamide
- ☐ B Erythromycin
- ☐ C Codeine
- ☐ D Amitriptyline
- ☐ E Magnesium

3.22 Amoxicillin is an appropriate first-line treatment for

- ☐ A acute otitis media
- ☐ B acute sore throat
- ☐ C suspected acute epiglottitis
- ☐ D sinusitis
- ☐ E mild bacterial chest infection

3.23 In renal failure dose reduction is required for

- ☐ A Captopril
- ☐ B Furosemide (frusemide)
- ☐ C Phenytoin
- ☐ D Cefuroxime
- ☐ E Gentamicin

3.24 The following drugs can precipitate attacks of acute intermittent porphyria (AIP):

☐ A Phenytoin
☐ B Rifampicin
☐ C Chlorpromazine
☐ D Griseofulvin
☐ E Aspirin

3.25 The following drugs may cause goitre:

☐ A Thyroxine
☐ B Iodine
☐ C Phenylbutazone
☐ D Lithium
☐ E Paracetamol

3.26 The following are recognised consequences of long-term use of topical steroids:

☐ A adrenal suppression
☐ B striae
☐ C vitiligo
☐ D skin malignancy
☐ E skin atrophy

3.27 Hormone replacement therapy (HRT) may

☐ A cause chloasma
☐ B cause hypocalcaemia
☐ C cause contact lens irritation
☐ D cause vaginal atrophy
☐ E provide a contraceptive effect

3.28 Gynaecomastia is a side-effect of the following drugs:

- ☐ A Cimetidine
- ☐ B Spironolactone
- ☐ C Ranitidine
- ☐ D Diethylstilbestrol
- ☐ E Amiodarone

3.29 The following are appropriate in the management of sickle cell crisis:

- ☐ A IM pethidine
- ☐ B IM morphine
- ☐ C Nitrous oxide
- ☐ D Oxygen
- ☐ E Antibiotics

3.30 The following drugs are teratogenic:

- ☐ A Warfarin
- ☐ B Phenytoin
- ☐ C Amoxicillin
- ☐ D Paracetamol
- ☐ E Carbimazole

3.31 The following can be used to treat a dry mouth:

- ☐ A Pilocarpine
- ☐ B Sugar-free chewing gum
- ☐ C Amitriptyline
- ☐ D Radiation
- ☐ E Artificial saliva

3.32 Ursodeoxycholic acid is:

- ☐ A   bile acid
- ☐ B   bile acid sequestrant
- ☐ C   used in the treatment of gallstones
- ☐ D   used in the treatment of primary biliary cirrhosis
- ☐ E   safe to use in pregnancy

3.33 Vitamin K must be given to a patient taking warfarin if

- ☐ A   there is major bleeding
- ☐ B   there is minor bleeding
- ☐ C   the international normalised ratio (INR) is greater than 8
- ☐ D   the INR is between 6 and 8
- ☐ E   the INR is between 5 and 6

3.34 The target INR should be 2.5 for:

- ☐ A   treatment of a deep vein thrombosis
- ☐ B   treatment of a pulmonary embolus
- ☐ C   atrial fibrillation
- ☐ D   mechanical prosthetic heart valve
- ☐ E   prosthetic heart valve replacement

3.35 The treatment of intermittent claudication includes

- ☐ A   stopping smoking
- ☐ B   reduction in daily exercise
- ☐ C   low-dose aspirin
- ☐ D   naftidrofuryl
- ☐ E   glyceryl trinitrate (GTN)

3.36 Zanamivir

☐ A should be given to all adults with influenza
☐ B should be given to at-risk adults when there is an epidemic of influenza
☐ C is only effective if given within the first 12 hours of symptoms
☐ D is given as an intravenous injection
☐ E is effective against influenza types A and B

3.37 The following are appropriate treatments for the respective viruses:

☐ A Ribovarin – respiratory syncytial virus (RSV)
☐ B Amantadine – influenza A
☐ C Aciclovir – herpes simplex
☐ D Alpha interferon – chronic hepatitis B
☐ E Ganciclovir – cytomegalovirus (CMV)

3.38 The following drugs are calcium-channel blockers:

☐ A Verapamil
☐ B Nifedipine
☐ C Nicorandil
☐ D Nimodipine
☐ E Nicardipine

3.39 The plasma concentration of sildenafil is altered by

☐ A Erythromycin
☐ B Antiviral drugs
☐ C Cimetidine
☐ D Ketoconazole
☐ E Grapefruit juice

3.40 The following drugs produce skeletal muscle relaxation by a direct effect on the muscle:

- ☐ A Dantroline
- ☐ B Baclofen
- ☐ C Diazepam
- ☐ D Tizanidine
- ☐ E Neostigmine

3.41 Alfacalcidol (1-alpha hydroxycholecalciferol) is

- ☐ A usually given by injection
- ☐ B metabolised to 1,25 dihydroxycholecalciferol
- ☐ C used to treat hypocalcaemia
- ☐ D a vitamin D derivative
- ☐ E used for osteoporosis

3.42 Regarding chemotherapy for colorectal cancer

- ☐ A fluorouracil is the mainstay of treatment
- ☐ B folinic acid should not be used
- ☐ C bone marrow suppression is a side-effect of fluorouracil
- ☐ D oxaliplatin may be used
- ☐ E drugs can be given IV or orally

3.43 In the treatment of breast cancer

- ☐ A tamoxifen is the treatment of choice
- ☐ B aminoglutethimide is an aromatase inhibitor
- ☐ C anastrozole is given pre-operatively as it is an aromatase inhibitor
- ☐ D chemotherapy is only used post-operatively
- ☐ E trastuzumab (Herceptin®) is used in metastatic disease

3.44 Tamoxifen

☐ A prevents breast cancer
☐ B protects against osteoporosis
☐ C causes thromboembolic events
☐ D causes endometrial cancer
☐ E causes hot flushes

3.45 The following may cause hyperprolactinaemia:

☐ A Metoclopramide
☐ B Chlorpropamide
☐ C Bromocriptine
☐ D L-dopa
☐ E Morphine

3.46 The yellow card system for adverse drug reactions

☐ A precisely estimates the frequency of side-effects
☐ B is used to report all reactions to established drugs
☐ C is used to report unusual or serious reactions to established drugs
☐ D is only used when a patient is taking several drugs
☐ E is sponsored by the pharmaceutical industry

3.47 Suppositories are useful as a mode of drug delivery because

☐ A drugs given by suppository do not cause nausea
☐ B they can be used to treat rectal disease locally
☐ C drugs absorbed from the rectum do not undergo first-pass metabolism in the liver
☐ D they rule out the side-effect of gastric irritation which occurs with oral diclofenac
☐ E they can be used to deliver drugs in patients who cannot swallow tablets

3.48 After 3 days' treatment with amoxicillin, a patient develops a red, macular, itchy rash. He

☐ A should never receive amoxicillin again
☐ B should never receive any penicillin again
☐ C can be treated safely with erythromycin
☐ D may be given flucloxacillin in the future
☐ E should avoid cefuroxime

3.49 Diabetes mellitus

☐ A can be treated with the biguanide metformin
☐ B can be treated with gliclazide which is short-acting
☐ C sulphonylureas decrease gluconeogenesis and peripheral utilisation of glucose
☐ D type 1 should be treated with glibenclamide
☐ E control is best maintained by testing the urine for glucose

3.50 Fluoxetine

☐ A is a monoamine-oxidase inhibitor
☐ B has an active metabolite
☐ C causes fewer antimuscarinic side-effects than tricyclic drugs
☐ D has a long half-life
☐ E may cause gastrointestinal haemorrhage

PAPER 3

Answers

The correct answer options for each question are given below.

3.1	A B E	3.26	A B E
3.2	A B D E F	3.27	A C
3.3	C	3.28	A B D
3.4	A B C	3.29	B D E
3.5	A B C D E	3.30	A B E
3.6	B C D	3.31	A B E
3.7	A C D	3.32	A C D
3.8	All false	3.33	A
3.9	A C	3.34	A B C
3.10	A D	3.35	A C D
3.11	A B C E	3.36	B E
3.12	A B E	3.37	A B C D E
3.13	A D E	3.38	A B D E
3.14	A D E	3.39	A B C D E
3.15	C D	3.40	A
3.16	C D	3.41	B C D E
3.17	A B E	3.42	A C D E
3.18	C D	3.43	B E
3.19	A B	3.44	A B C D E
3.20	B	3.45	A
3.21	A C D	3.46	C
3.22	A D E	3.47	B E
3.23	A D E	3.48	D
3.24	A B D	3.49	A B
3.25	C D	3.50	B C D E

Paper 3

Answers and teaching notes

3.1 Adverse effects of ACE inhibitors include   Answers: A B E

Side-effects include taste disturbance, rashes, neutropenia, proteinuria. Dry cough is common. It is used to treat the hypertension. First-dose hypotension is an important side-effect, especially in patients with heart failure where loop diuretics are also being used. Captopril is used for hypertension, cardiac failure, post-myocardial infarction, diabetic nephropathy and progressive renal failure but not in renal artery stenosis.

3.2 Isoniazid   Answers: A B D E F

Isoniazid is given in two phases:

• 2 months → isoniazid + rifampicin + pyrazinamide
• next 4 months → isoniazid + rifampicin

Isoniazid is metabolised in the liver by acetylation. This depends on genetic factors (some people are 'fast' acetylators and others are 'slow' acetylators). Side-effects include skin rashes, hepatotoxicity and blood dyscrasias and peripheral neuritis with high doses. Peripheral neuropathy is due to a deficiency in pyridoxine and this is prevented by giving pyridoxine prophylactically. Isoniazid is excreted renally. It decreases the metabolism of phenytoin and carbamazepine, resulting in an increase in plasma levels and toxicity. Rapid acetylators have lower drug concentrations, and therefore experience a higher rate of relapse.

3.3 Captopril   Answer: C

Captopril is an ACE inhibitor:

Angiotensin I

$\downarrow$ ACE   captopril inhibits this

Angiotensin II
(Vasoconstrictor)

Vasodilatation results in first-dose hypotension. A cough is a common side-effect. Patients with heart failure are likely to experience more hypotension and first-dose hypotension than hypertensive patients.

3.4 Left ventricular failure (LVF)   Answers: A B C

The first-line treatment of LVF is oxygen (100%), diuretics, e.g. furosemide (frusemide) or bendroflumethiazide (bendrofluazide) and ACE inhibitors, e.g. enalapril. Dobutamine has an inotropic effect. Diamorphine causes vasodilatation. 200J DC shock is used in cardiac arrest with asystole. IV adrenaline (epinephrine) is used in asystole. Although it increases cardiac contractility it is also a potent vasoconstrictor. Other drugs – digoxin increases the force of contraction of the heart. In heart failure, it is used in patients who have atrial fibrillation or whose symptoms are not relieved by diuretics and ACE inhibitors. Nitrates, e.g. GTN are vasodilators which reduce pre-load and are used for symptomatic relief in acute LVF.

3.5 Thiazide diuretics   Answers: A B C D E

Thiazides are used to treat chronic heart failure and mild hypertension. They inhibit Na^+ reabsorption in the distal convoluted tubule. Metabolic effects are uncommon in low dose, but can include:

- hypercalcaemia
- hyperglycaemia
- hyperuricaemia
- hypomagnesaemia
- hypercholesterolaemia
- hyponatraemia
- hypocalcaemia

3.6 Carbimazole   Answers: B C D

Carbimazole is a pro-drug converted to methimazole. It can cause agranulocytosis in the first 3 months of therapy, and patients should be advised to report a sore throat or mouth ulcers. Radioactive iodine is contraindicated in pregnancy. Carbimazole or propylthiouracil can be used in pregnancy but carbimazole may cause fetal goitre and should be used with care. Carbimazole inhibits thyroid hormone production. Propylthiouracil inhibits conversion of T_4 to T_3.

3.7 Sodium cromoglicate   Answers: A C D

Regular inhalation of sodium cromoglicate is used to decrease the incidence of asthma attacks. It is used for prophylaxis and is of no value in an acute attack.

In general it is more effective in adults than children and in adults it allows dose reduction of bronchodilators and oral corticosteroids.

It is difficult to determine who will benefit and it is reasonable to try it for a period of 4 to 6 weeks. Treatment with sodium cromoglicate involves daily inhalation with frequency adjusted according to response but is usually three to four times daily.

Sodium cromoglicate is of value in the prevention of exercise-induced asthma; a single dose is given 30 minutes before exercise.

Inhalation of the dry powder form may cause bronchospasm and if this occurs a selective β_2-stimulant such as salbutamol should be inhaled a few minutes beforehand.

3.8 Leukotriene receptor antagonists   Answers: All false

Leukotrienes have a constrictor effect on the bronchi and leukotriene receptor antagonists have been developed to block this effect. They are used in the prophylaxis of asthma and should not be used to relieve an attack of acute severe asthma.

Using a leukotriene receptor antagonist does not necessarily allow a reduction in existing corticosteroid treatment and care should be taken if withdrawal of steroids is contemplated. Side-effects include hypersensitivity reactions, including anaphylaxis. Churg–Strauss syndrome has also been reported. Currently, the new leukotriene receptor inhibitors are administered in tablet form. The leukotriene receptor antagonists include montelukast and zafirlukast.

3.9 Drugs that act on the CNS   Answers: A C

Most anti-emetics have a sedating effect via their action on the CNS. Domperidone, however, does not cross the blood–brain barrier, and exerts its effect by increasing gastric emptying. In Parkinson's disease, treatment is aimed at increasing levels of dopamine in the CNS. Levodopa is converted to dopamine, by dopa decarboxylase, both centrally and peripherally, but the peripheral action of dopamine causes unwanted side-effects.

A peripheral decarboxylase inhibitor prevents conversion of levodopa to dopamine peripherally so that more levodopa can cross the blood–brain barrier. Benserazide and carbidopa are both peripheral dopa-decarboxylase inhibitors.

3.10 Drugs for the treatment of Alzheimer's disease   Answers: A D

The cholinesterase-inhibiting drugs, donepezil and rivastigmine are used in the treatment of mild to moderate Alzheimer's disease. Improvement is assessed by cognitive testing 3 months after starting treatment. The drugs are given orally. Drug treatment should only be initiated and supervised by a dementia specialist.

3.11 Benzodiazepines   Answers: A B C E

Benzodiazepines are used for their sedative effect, alleviation of anxiety and production of amnesia. These properties make them useful as premedication for general anaesthesia. Benzodiazepines have an antiepileptic action and diazepam is used in the treatment of status epilepticus. Benzodiazepines have no analgesic effects, and are ineffective in the treatment of depression, psychosis and phobic states. An important side-effect of benzodepines is respiratory depression, which can be reversed by flumazenil.

3.12 Bleeding from the GI tract   Answers: A B E

All non-steroidal anti-inflammatory drugs (NSAIDs) may cause GI bleeding. Rofecoxib and celecoxib, selective cyclo-oxygenase-2 inhibitors have fewer GI side-effects and they are licensed for symptomatic relief in osteoarthritis. Celecoxib is also licensed for the relief of pain and inflammation in rheumatoid arthritis. Ferrous sulphate may cause bleeding, especially in overdose. Lansoprazole is a proton pump inhibitor and is used to treat ulcers. Aminophylline can cause gastric irritation.

3.13 Asthma   Answers: A D E

Prostaglandins such as prostacyclin produce bronchodilation, and aspirin inhibits prostaglandin synthesis, exacerbating asthma. Aspirin does this in 96% of asthmatics. In 2% there is no effect and 2% improve. Aspirin is related to tartrazine (a food colouring in orange squash etc.) and patients with asthma should also avoid tartrazine. Corticosteroids induce synthesis of lipocortin, which inhibits phospholipase A_2. In addition, corticosteroids inhibit the production of cytokines, which has a pro-inflammatory effect. Codeine phosphate and diazepam cause respiratory depression and therefore may reduce respiratory function. Occasionally, if a patient with asthma is suffering from a cough with bronchospasm, codeine may be useful, but this should be used with caution.

3.14 Analgesics   Answers: A D E

Analgesics are more effective in preventing pain than treating established pain. Non-steroidal anti-inflammatory drugs are highly effective analgesics and often, used correctly, make opioids unnecessary. Morphine and diamorphine may be given orally, subcutaneously or intravenously, but the greater solubility of diamorphine allows smaller volumes to be injected; this is an advantage in an emaciated patient. Fentanyl, alfentanil and remifentanil are used by injection for intra-operative analgesia and fentanyl may also be administered by the transdermal route as a patch.

3.15 Healing of a peptic ulcer   Answers: C D

H_2-blockers such as ranitidine decrease gastric acid production and allow healing of an ulcer. Chlorphenamine (chlorpheniramine) is an H_1-receptor blocker. Bismuth has anti-*Helicobacter* properties. There is no evidence that spicy food increases the risk of ulceration or that non-spicy food allows healing. Rest may help heal stress-induced ulceration.

3.16 Lipid-lowering drugs   Answers: C D

Lowering the concentration of low density lipoprotein (LDL) cholesterol and raising high density lipoprotein (HDL) cholesterol reduces the progression of coronary atherosclerosis and may even induce regression.

There is evidence that if LDL cholesterol can be lowered by 25% to 35%, primary and secondary prevention of coronary heart disease is achieved. Treatment with statins has been shown to reduce myocardial infarction, coronary deaths and overall mortality.

Statins are drugs of first choice for treating hypercholesterolaemia; fibrates for treating hypertriglyceridaemia; and statins or fibrates can be used either together, or alone, to treat mixed hyperlipidaemia.

Rhabdomyolysis associated with lipid-regulating drugs such as the fibrates and statins is rare – approximately one case in every 100,000 treatment-years.

3.17 Antibiotic prophylaxis   Answers: A B E

Antibiotic prophylaxis to prevent endocarditis is needed in patients with cardiac valvular prosthesis or disease, septal defects or previous endocarditis. For tonsillectomy and bronchoscopy, ampicillin and gentamicin should be given intramuscularly 1 hour before the procedure. For sigmoidoscopy, the same applies but amoxicillin (500 mg) should additionally be taken 6 hours after the procedure. Cystoscopy, catheterisation, D&C, labour and IUCD removal/insertion only require antibiotic prophylaxis if there is a urinary tract infection, in which case the antibiotics should be appropriate for the infective organism. Note that if the patient is allergic to penicillin or has had more than two courses in the last month, vancomycin should be given instead of ampicillin.

3.18 Meningitis   Answers: C D

If the diagnosis of meningitis is suspected, blood cultures should be taken and a decision made on the need for a CT scan before performing lumbar puncture. The incidence of complications increases with a delay in starting antibiotic treatment. Pneumococcal meningitis is best treated with high doses of cephalosporin. Meningococcal meningitis should be initially treated with IV benzylpenicillin (2.4 g six times a day). *Haemophilus* meningitis can be treated with cefotaxime IV (2 g t.d.s.) (or in children ceftriaxone IV). Contacts also need to be traced and treated. Meningitis caused by *listeria* is treated with ampicillin and gentamicin. If the organism is unknown, cefotaxime should be given to adults; ampicillin and cefotaxime are preferred in children or immunocompromised adults.

3.19 Trimethoprim   Answers: A B

Specimens should be taken for culture and sensitivities before starting treatment. Therapy can be changed later when the results are known. In a non-pregnant woman presenting with a first episode of cystitis, a suitable antibiotic treatment is trimethoprim or amoxicillin or nitrofurantoin. If the initial treatment fails, cefradine or ciprofloxacin should be prescribed. Prostatitis can be treated with trimethoprin, ciprofloxacin or erythromycin, which have good tissue penetration. Epididymo-orchitis is treated with ciprofloxacin. Pyelonephritis can be initially treated with cefotaxime, gentamicin and treatment modified according to microbiological findings. Atrophic vaginitis is related to oestrogen deficiency occurring around or after the menopause and can be treated with hormone cream.

3.20 Gastric lavage   Answer: B

Gastric lavage and single-dose activated charcoal are used to prevent absorption of drugs from the stomach in cases of overdose/
poisoning. Iron and lithium are not absorbed by activated charcoal
and gastric lavage is used. Gastric lavage is contraindicated in
ingestion of hydrocarbons and corrosives (e.g. caustic soda). Lavage
should not be undertaken if the patient has a depressed conscious
level unless the airway is protected by a cuffed endotracheal tube,
and is also contraindicated if the patient is at risk of a gastric
haemorrhage or perforation.

3.21 Constipation   Answers: A C D

Constipation, i.e. increased gut transit time, is caused by sympathetic nervous system activation, parasympathetic nervous system inhibition (e.g. by anticholinergics and antidepressants), opiates, and
aluminium salts.

Diarrhoea, i.e. reduced gut transit time, is a side-effect of magnesium
salts; antibiotics may cause pseudomembranous colitis; erythromycin also causes diarrhoea due to a pro-kinetic effect on the gut.

3.22 Amoxicillin   Answers: A D E

Amoxicillin is appropriate first-line treatment for acute otitis media,
sinusitis, and mild lobar pneumonia. If a patient is allergic to penicillin, erythromycin is a suitable alternative. Acute streptococcal sore
throat should be treated with penicillin. Acute epiglottitis should be
treated with cefotaxime in adults, or ceftriaxone in children.

3.23 Renal failure   Answers: A D E

When captopril is administered, toxicity may occur if creatinine
clearance is low. ACE inhibitors are contraindicated in renal artery
stenosis. Furosemide (frusemide) acts on the loop of Henle in the
nephron: if the number of functioning nephrons decreases (i.e. in
renal failure) there are fewer loops of Henle on which it can exert its
diuretic effect and the dose may need to be increased. Phenytoin is

metabolised by the liver and largely protein-bound in the blood. Most cephalosporins are excreted unchanged by the kidney and therefore accumulate in renal failure. A reduction in dose frequency is usually necessary. Gentamicin is excreted by the kidney and is nephrotoxic; close therapeutic dose monitoring is required.

3.24 Acute intermittent porphyria   Answers: A B D

There is a long list of drugs that can cause AIP. It is worth knowing the common ones which include: oral contraceptives, barbiturates, alcohol, cephalosporins, phenytoin and rifampicin.

3.25 Goitre   Answers: C D

A goitre is an enlarged thyroid gland. The thyroid hypertrophies under the influence if TSH which is secreted by the anterior pituitary in response to T3 and T4. If T3 and T4 production by the thyroid falls, then TSH rises and the thyroid gland is stimulated. Drugs that decrease the synthesis and release of T3 and T4 will cause an increase in TSH production and this may result in a goitre, whereas exogenous thyroxine will decrease TSH. Iodine is needed for thyroid hormone production and a deficiency may lead to a goitre.

Phenylbutazone is a non-steroidal anti-inflammatory drug that is used in the treatment of ankylosing spondylitis. It has many other side-effects, including parotitis, pancreatitis, hepatitis, nephritis and visual disturbances. Lithium may cause hypothyroidism and goitre. It inhibits the release of the thyroid hormones form the gland itself. Paracetamol does not affect thyroid hormone production.

3.26 Topical steroids   Answers: A B E

Steroids, when applied directly to the skin, can cause skin atrophy. Local vascular changes may occur, producing purpura and striae. Vitiligo is a systemic condition, producing areas of depigmentation, usually at multiple sites. Topical steroids do not increase the risk of skin malignancy.

3.27 HRT
Answers: A C

Side-effects of HRT include nausea and vomiting, premenstrual type symptoms, liver dysfunction, migraine, depression, and contact lens irritation. Vaginal atrophy is treated by HRT (topical creams are usually sufficient). HRT does not provide contraception. Women are considered potentially fertile for 2 years after the last menstrual period if under 50 years old, and for 1 year if older than 50.

3.28 Gynaecomastia
Answers: A B D

Gynaecomastia is caused by:

* Oestrogen
* Prolactin stimulants
* Other drugs such as cimetidine, digoxin and spironolactone
* Cimetidine is an H_2 antagonist, which also exerts its action at androgen receptors. Other H_2 antagonists do not have the same effect
* Digoxin – on long-term use
* Spironolactone
* Methyldopa
* Diethylstilbestrol is an oestrogen preparation occasionally used to treat breast cancer. It causes gynaecomastia in men.

3.29 Sickle cell crisis
Answers: B D E

Morphine should be given as soon as possible, oxygen administered at 4 l/min is useful in compromised patients. In the presence of an infection/fever an antibiotic such as cefotaxime is suitable. Pethidine should not be given as it is associated with grand mal seizures in certain patients. Nitrous oxide should not be administered as it can cause acute irreversible neuropathy.

3.30 Teratogenic drugs
Answers: A B E

Warfarin produces congenital malformations. Phenytoin produces congenital malformations – folate is given to the mother to prevent this. Penicillins are not harmful. Antibiotics are needed to treat UTIs in pregnancy – Amoxil® and cefalexin are suitable. Paracetamol is used safely in pregnancy. Carbimazole causes neonatal goitre and hypothyroidism. Drugs which are teratogenic include: alcohol, warfarin, phenytoin and other anticonvulsants, lithium, progestogens and androgens.

3.31 Dry mouth   Answers: A B E

Dry mouth (xerostomia) may be caused by drugs with anticholinergic side-effects, such as tricyclic antidepressants, and irradiation, e.g. for treatment for head and neck cancers. Sjögren's syndrome causes dryness of the eye and mouth. Simple measures often relieve symptoms in many patients, e.g. frequent sips of cool drinks, ice or sugar-free pastilles. Sugar-free chewing gum stimulates salivation in patients with residual salivary function. Artificial saliva can provide useful relief and many preparations are available. Pilocarpine tablets are licensed for the treatment of xerostomia following irradiation of the head and neck and for a dry mouth and dry eyes caused by Sjögren's syndrome.

3.32 Ursodeoxycholic acid   Answers: A C D

Ursodeoxycholic acid is a bile acid that can be used to treat gallstone disease in patients not able to undergo a surgical procedure, if symptoms are mild, there is normal gallbladder function, and small- or medium-sized radiolucent stones. It is not suitable for radio-opaque stones, which are unlikely to dissolve. Patients should also be given appropriate dietary advice (cholesterol and calorie reduction). Gallstones may recur in up to 25% of patients within 1 year of having treatment. Ursodeoxycholic acid is also used for primary biliary cirrhosis. Liver tests improve in most patients but an overall increase in survival has not been demonstrated. A bile acid sequestrant forms an insoluble complex with the bile acids, relieving diarrhoea and pruritus. An example of this is colestyramine which is useful in the management of primary biliary cirrhosis to relieve the pruritus and in Crohn's disease to decrease diarrhoea.

Ursodeoxycholic acid is contraindicated in pregnancy. It is also contraindicated where the enterohepatic circulation of bile salts is disrupted as in inflammatory bowel disease and other conditions of the small intestine and colon. Side-effects of ursodeoxycholic acid include nausea, vomiting, diarrhoea and pruritus.

3.33 Vitamin K   Answer: A

The following recommendations are based on the British Society for Haematology Guidelines and are based on the result of the INR and whether there is major or minor bleeding. The recommendations for patients taking warfarin are:

Major bleeding – stop warfarin and give vitamin K, 5 mg by slow IV injection. In addition, a prothrombin complex concentrate (factors II, VII, IX and X) or fresh frozen plasma should be given.

If the INR is greater than 8 and there is minor bleeding or no bleeding warfarin should be stopped and restarted when the INR falls below 5. If there are other risk factors for bleeding then vitamin K, 0.5 mg should be given by slow intravenous injection or 5 mg by mouth. The dose may be repeated if the INR is still too high after 24 hours.

If the INR is between 6 and 8 and there is no bleeding or minor bleeding warfarin should be stopped and restarted when the INR is less than 5.

If the INR is less than 6 but more than 0.5 units above the target value warfarin should be stopped or the dose reduced and restarted when the INR is less than 5.

If the INR is at therapeutic levels but there is unexpected bleeding then the possibility of underlying disease of the renal or GI tract should be investigated.

3.34 Target INR   Answers: A B C

The indications and target INRs currently recommended by the British Society of Haematology are: INR 2–2.5 for the prophylaxis of deep vein thrombosis. INR 2.5: for the treatment of deep vein thrombosis and pulmonary embolism, atrial fibrillation, cardioversion, dilated cardiomyopathy, mural thrombus following myocardial infarction and rheumatic mitral valve disease. INR 3.5: for recurrent deep vein thrombosis, pulmonary embolism, metallic prosthetic valves, or if thromboembolic disease recurs when patients are already receiving warfarin to a target INR of 2.5. (Porcine valve replacement patients do not require anticoagulation.)

3.35 Treatment of intermittent claudication   Answers: A C D

The most important measures in the conservative management of intermittent claudication include stopping smoking and increased exercise with a training programme. Low-dose aspirin should be given as a long-term prophylactic against cardiovascular events and a statin should be considered if serum total cholesterol is raised. Naftidrofuryl may alleviate symptoms and improve pain-free walking distance in moderate disease. It is not known whether it has any effect on the outcome of the disease. GTN is a potent coronary artery dilator but its main effect is as a peripheral veno-dilator. It relieves angina by decreasing the venous return and therefore the workload of the heart. As it is a peripheral veno-dilator it will not help symptoms of intermittent claudication which is due to occlusion of peripheral arteries.

3.36 Zanamivir: Answers: B E

Zanamivir is licensed for the treatment of influenza A or B within 48 hours after the onset of symptoms. In other words, healthy individuals. It reduces the duration of symptoms by about 1 day. It is given by inhalation of powder. Care must be taken with patients with asthma as there is a risk of bronchospasm.

The National Institute for Clinical Excellence (NICE) has issued guidance for the use of Zanamivir for the treatment of influenza. The recommendations are:

* Zanamivir should not be used to treat otherwise healthy adults with influenza.
* Zanamivir should be used to treat at-risk adults when influenza is circulating in the community if they are able to commence treat-

95

ment within 48 hours of the onset of symptoms.

At-risk patients are defined as those over 65 years of age or those who have one or more of the following conditions:

- chronic respiratory disease (but care should be taken because of the risk of bronchospasm)
- significant cardiovascular disease (but not hypertension)
- immunosuppression
- diabetes mellitus.

The guidance does not cover the circumstance of an pandemic or widespread epidemic of a new strain of influenza to which there is little or no community resistance.

3.37 Antiviral drugs   Answers: A B C D E

Ribavirin inhibits a wide range of DNA and RNA viruses. It is given by inhalation for the treatment of severe bronchiolitis caused by RSV in infants. Ribavirin is given by mouth with interferon alpha-2b for the treatment of chronic hepatitis C infection. It is also effective in Lassa fever.

Amantadine may be used for prophylaxis during an outbreak of influenza A in certain at-risk groups. Aciclovir is effective in herpes simplex and varicella but does not eradicate the virus. It is effective only if started at the onset of the infection. Interferon alpha is used in the treatment of chronic hepatitis B but its success is limited by a response rate of less than 50%. Interferon alpha is also used in the treatment of chronic hepatitis C. Ganciclovir is used in the treatment of cytomegalovirus. Foscarnet is also active against cytomegalovirus but is toxic and can cause renal impairment. Cidofovir can be used for CMV retinitis in AIDS patients if ganciclovir and foscarnet are contraindicated.

3.38 Calcium-channel blockers   Answers: A B D E

Calcium-channel blockers interfere with the inward displacement of calcium ions through the slow channels of active cell membranes. They may affect the myocardial cells and the cells within the specialised conducting system of the heart. Calcium-channel blockers also affect the cells of vascular smooth muscle. Verapamil is used for the treatment of angina, hypertension and arrhythmias, and is a highly negative inotropie (calcium-channel blocker) and reduces cardiac output and heart rate. It may precipitate heart failure and should not be used with β-blockers. Dihydropyridine calcium-channel blockers, e.g. nifedipine, affect vascular smooth muscle more than cardiac tissue. (Nifedepine relaxes vascular smooth muscle and dilates coronary and peripheral arteries.) They do not produce clinical deterioration in heart failure, and are used for angina of hypertension and are valuable in forms of angina associated with coronary vaso-spasm. Nimodipine is related to nifedipine but its smooth muscle relaxant effect acts preferentially on the cerebral arteries. Its use is confined to prevention of cardiovascular spasm following subarachnoid haemorrhage. Nicorandil is a potassium-channel activator used in the prophylaxis and treatment of angina.

3.39 Sildenafil   Answers: A B C D E

Erythromycin, itraconazole and ketoconazole, many antivirals and cimetidine increase plasma sildenafil concentration. Grapefruit juice may also increase plasma concentration! Care should also be taken to avoid concomitant use with nicorandil as the hypotensive effect is significantly enhanced (and nitrates for the same reason).

3.40 Skeletal muscle relaxation   Answer: A

Dantroline acts directly on skeletal muscle and produces few essential adverse effects making it a drug of choice. Baclofen inhibits transmission at spinal level and also depresses the CNS. Diazepam mainly acts centrally and sedation is an important side-effect. Tizanidine is a newly introduced α_2-adrenoreceptor agonist and is indicated for spasticity associated with multiple sclerosis or spinal cord injury. Neostigmine enhances neuromuscular transmission resulting in enhanced muscular contraction and not relaxation as stated in the question.

3.41 Alfacalcidol   Answers: B C D E

Alfacalcidol is a vitamin D derivative.
Vitamin D consists of:
Ergocalciferol = vitamin D2
Colecalciferol = vitamin D3
Alfacalcidol = 1-alpha hydroxycholecalciferol
Calcitriol = 1,25-dihydroxycholecalciferol
1-alpha hydroxycholecalciferol is hydroxylated by the kidney to the active form.
1,25-dihydroxycholecalciferol. Vitamin D deficiency is caused by liver disease, intestinal malabsorption or hypoparathyroidism will cause hypocalcaemia, which requires administration of vitamin D orally. There is a resultant risk of hypercalcaemia and levels should be measured regularly. Osteoporosis can be treated with vitamin D supplementation.

3.42 Chemotherapy for colorectal cancer   Answers: A C D E

Fluorouracil is a pro-drug that is converted to metabolites that inhibit thymidylate synthetase, thereby preventing DNA synthesis. It is the mainstay of drug therapy for colorectal cancer. The addition of folinic acid potentiates the effect of fluorouracil and forms part of the standard first-line treatment. Fluorouracil is toxic on gut mucosa and bone marrow, causing colitis, mucositis and gastritis. Less common effects are alopecia, nail changes and photosensitivity.

Oxaliplatin is a platinum compound that is used with fluorouracil or folinic acid for metastatic colorectal cancer.

Oral formulations of fluoropyrimidines are more convenient for patients than IV treatment and avoid the need for intravascular catheters. Oral medication is as effective as IV regimes.

3.43 Treatment of breast cancer   Answers: B E

Breast cancer is treated primarily by surgery. Endocrine treatments such as tamoxifen and the aromatase inhibitors are used as adjuvant therapy.

Their main benefits are the prevention of recurrence and prevention of a second tumour in the contralateral breast. In some patients not suitable for surgery, endocrine therapy may be used as primary therapy to suppress tumour growth.

Aromatase inhibitors such as anastrozole and letrozole inhibit peripheral synthesis of oestrogen. They may be used (occasionally) pre-operatively but this is **not** because of their action as aromatase inhibitors.

Aminoglutethimide is a non-steroidal aromatase inhibitor. Chemotherapy can be used pre-operatively (neoadjuvant therapy) to downstage tumours. Post-operative chemotherapy is used to treat metastases. Herceptin® is a monoclonal antibody used in the management of metastatic disease.

3.44 Tamoxifen   Answers: A B C D E

Tamoxifen is a partial agonist, i.e. both agonist and antagonist. Due to its action as an oestrogen-receptor antagonist, it is used as an adjuvant hormonal treatment in patients with oestrogen-receptor-positive breast cancer. It should be continued for 5 years.

The oestrogen agonist effects account for its other actions and side-effects. These are prevention of osteoporosis and a decrease in cholesterol levels. Tamoxifen has oestrogenic effects on the uterus, increasing the risk of endometrial cancer. Tamoxifen increases the risk of thromboembolic events.

3.45 Hyperprolactinaemia   Answer: A

Metoclopramide acts on the chemoreceptor trigger zone to stimulate gastric motility and is used as an anti-emetic. Chlorpropamide is easily confused with chlorpromazine. Chlorpromazine is an antipsychotic drug. Actions include:
• a block of dopamine receptors, causing hyperprolactinaemia and galactorrhoea
• extrapyramidal effects such as parkinsonian symptoms, akathisia, tardive dyskinesia

- antimuscarinic effects – dry mouth, constipation, blurred vision, micturition difficulty
- cardiovascular effects – hypotension, tachycardia, arrhythmias
- sensitivity reactions – agranulocytosis, leucopenia, haemolytic anaemia, photosensitisation.

Bromocriptine stimulates dopamine receptors in the brain. Prolactin secretion by the pituitary is inhibited by dopamine:

$$\text{Dopamine} \longrightarrow \begin{array}{c} \text{Pituitary} \\ \downarrow \\ \text{Prolactin} \end{array}$$

Bromocriptine also inhibits growth hormone secretion. L-dopa is a precursor of dopamine.

3.46 The yellow card system   Answer: C

This is a reporting system on side-effects and reactions to drugs. No precise numbers are required. All reactions to new drugs should be reported. Unusual and serious reactions to all drugs should be reported. The yellow card system of adverse drug reactions is appropriate for all patients, however many drugs are being taken. It is conducted by the Committee on Safety of Medicines.

3.47 Suppositories   Answers: B E

Suppositories are used to deliver medication via the rectum. The rectum has a rich blood supply and therefore is able to absorb drugs into the blood stream rapidly. The side-effects therefore do occur, including nausea.

Rectal administration is useful for topical therapy of steroids for proctitis and colitis, in the form of suppositories or foam enema.

Drugs absorbed in the rectum into the bloodstream undergo hepatic metabolism in the usual way.

Rectal administration of diclofenac does not rule out the side-effect of gastric irritation or ulceration. In patients who cannot swallow tablets or who are deliberately made 'nil by mouth', rectal administration is very useful.

3.48 Macular, itchy rash   Answer: D

A patient who develops a rash following amoxicillin treatment may not necessarily be allergic to the amoxicillin. The danger of anaphylaxis relates to a second dose of a drug after sensitisation by the first dose and this patient has already had 3 days of treatment.

Patients who are truly allergic to penicillin should be treated with erythromycin where antibiotic therapy is required. However, erythromycin may also cause a reaction in itself and therefore cannot be deemed to be entirely safe.

Flucloxacillin is a penicillin derivative and may be used.

Cephalosporin sensitivity is seen in approximately 10% of penicillin-allergic patients.

3.49 Diabetes mellitus   Answers: A B

Oral antidiabetic medication is used to treat type 2 diabetes mellitus. This is non-insulin-dependent diabetes. The sulphonylureas act by increasing insulin secretion. Long-acting ones include chlorpropamide and glibenclamide. Short-acting examples are gliclazide and tolbutamide. Metformin is the only biguanide. It decreases gluconeogenesis and increases peripheral glucose utilisation. Metformin can be used with sulphonylureas. Metformin may cause lactic acidosis in patients with renal impairment. Control is best maintained by checking blood sugar levels.

Other antidiabetics include:

- acarbose which delays the digestion and absorption of starch
- guar gum, which reduces postprandial plasma glucose
- nateglinide and repaglinide, which stimulate insulin relase
- pioglitazone and rosiglitazone, which reduce peripheral insulin resistance.

3.50 Fluoxetine   Answers: B C D E

Fluoxetine is a selective serotonin inhibitor (SSRI) used in the treatment of depression. SSRIs are less sedating and have fewer anticholinergic side-effects than tricylic antidepressants. The side-effects include GI effects such as nausea, vomiting, diarrhoea, and bleeding. Fluoxetine has a long half-life with a long duration of action. When changing antidepressant medication, monoamine oxidase inhibitors (MAOIs) should not be started for at least 5 weeks after stopping fluoxetine.

Index

INDEX

penicillin 2, 7, 8, 17, 24, 25, 73,
81, 89, 101
peptic ulcers 8, 17, 25, 46, 56, 65,
72, 88
peripheral neuropathy 41, 57
pethidine 76, 92
phaeochromocytoma 42, 58
pharmcokinetic variation 9, 27
phenoxybenzamine 42, 58
phenylbutazone 75, 91
phenytoin 4, 13, 20, 31, 32, 38, 54,
74, 75, 76, 90, 92
photosensitivity 35, 50
pituitary ablation 36
pizotifen 43, 60
potassium chloride 40, 56
prednisolone 8, 10, 25, 29, 31, 40,
55
prednisone 12, 31
pregnancy, as contraindication 77,
93
prescriptions 47, 66
pro-drugs 12, 31, 44, 61, 70, 85
probenecid 12, 31
prochlorperazine 42, 58
progesterone 26
progestogen 41, 43, 57, 59–60
promethazine 45, 64
propranolol 10, 12, 28, 31, 40, 47,
55, 66
propylthiouracil 84
prostaglandins 87
prostatis 7, 89
proton pump inhibitors 17
pseudocholinesterase deficiency 9,
27
psoriasis 12, 30
pyelonephritis 73, 89
pyridoxine 69, 83

ranitidine 8, 13, 25, 31, 46, 65, 72,
88
reactions to drugs 46, 65, 80, 81,
100
reflux oesophagitis 2, 17
renal failure 3, 19, 21, 35, 50, 74,
90
respiratory depression 87

respiratory syncytial virus (RSV) 78,
96
resuscitation 11, 29
rhabdomyolysis 73, 88
ribovarin 78
rifampicin 5, 13, 22, 32, 39, 41, 55,
57, 75, 83, 91
riluzole 47, 66
rivastigmine 86

sacralfate 8, 25
salbutamol 8, 12, 16, 25, 44, 62
salmeterol 12, 31, 44, 62
scabies 12, 30
sedation 72, 86
selegiline 1, 3, 16, 19, 39, 55
senna 8, 25
shingles 44, 61
sickle cell 42, 58, 76, 92
sigmoidoscopy 73, 88
sildenafil 47, 66, 78, 97
simvastin 11, 29
sinusitis 74, 90
Sjögren's syndrome 93
skeletal muscle relaxation 79, 97
smoking 41, 57, 77, 95
sodium 41, 57
sodium cromoglycate 71, 85
sore throat 74, 90
spironolactone 5, 22, 76, 92
statins 73, 88, 95
steroids, topical 75, 91
stress, and blood sugar 64
striae 75, 91
stroke 11, 30, 49
prevention 8, 26
sulphasalazine 8, 25
sulphonamides 38, 54
sumatriptan 43, 60
suppositories 80, 100
surgery, drugs stopped before 44,
62
suxamethorium 37, 52

tachycardia 10, 13, 28, 32
tamoxifen 79, 80, 98, 99
tartrazine 87
taste disturbance 69, 83

107

PASTEST BOOKS FOR MEDICAL STUDENTS

The Practical Guide to Medical Ethics and Law for Junior Doctors and Medical Students

M Brennan, C Baxter, Y Coldicott

- Excellent guidance on how to study ethics and law
- Practical guidance on how to pass your exams
- Real case studies from international doctors
- Top tips based on real life incidents

Clinical Skills for Medical Students: A Hands-on Guide

Bickle, Hamilton, et al

- Covers system-based chapter i.e. cardiovascular, respiratory with other common examinations
- Useful tips on how to write-up and present a case including case history
- Clear diagrams to explain difficult concepts

Radiology Casebook for Medical Students

R Wasan, A Grundy, R Beese

- Covers X-rays, MR and CT scans
- Read our guidance section to enhance your interpretation skills
- Take the test paper to confirm you are on the right track

EMQs for Medical Students Volumes 1 & 2

A Feather et al

Two volumes of EMQs covering all major themes. Written by doctors at the forefront of medical education with invaluable experience in writing best-sellers for medical students.

- Cover all topics likely to be assessed during medical training
- Over 100 themes contained in each volume
- Essential list of normal values

OSCEs for Medical Undergraduates Volumes 1 & 2
R Visvanathan, A Feather JSP Lumley
Volume 1 *covers*: Cardiovascular Diseases, Neurology, Psychiatry, Ophthalmology, Otolaryngology, Haematology, respiratory Medicine, Orthopaedics, Trauma, Ethics and Legal Medicine.
Volume 2 *covers*: Endocrinology, Gastroenterology, Urology, Renal Medicine, Obstetrics, Gynaecology, Rheumatology and Dermatology.
Each book covers:
- History taking, clinical examinations, investigations, practical techniques, making a diagnosis, prescribing treatment and other issues
- Answers and additional information so that you can assess your performance and identify areas needing further attention
- Contain X-rays, scans, haematological and biochemical results and a colour slide section

Surgical Finals: Passing the Clinical
Kuperberg & Lumley
- 90 examples of favourite long and short surgical cases
- Syllabus checklist for structured revision
- 18 detailed examination schemes with action tables
- 36 tables of differential diagnosis
- 134 popular viva questions for self-assessment
- Recommended reading list and revision index

Medical Finals: Passing the Clinical
Moore & Richardson
- 101 typical long cases, short cases and spot diagnoses
- Syllabus checklist for systematic revision
- Vital tips on preparation and presentation
- Structured examination plans for all cases
- Concise teaching notes highlight areas most relevant to finals
- Revision index for easy access to specific topics

Surgical Finals: Structured Answer and Essay Questions
Visvanathan & Lumley
- Prepare for the written examination with this unique combination of essay questions and the new structured answer questions
- 111 structured answer questions with detailed teaching notes

- 52 typical essay questions with sample essay plans and model essays
- Invaluable revision checklist to help you to trach your progress
- Short textbook reviews enable you to select the best textbooks

Medical Finals: Structured Answer and Essay Questions
Feather, Visvanathan & Lumley
- Prepare for the written examination with this unique combination of essay questions and the new structured answer questions
- 141 structured answer questions with detailed teaching notes
- 73 typical essay questions with sample essay plans and model essays
- Invaluable revision checklist to help you to trach your progress
- Short textbook reviews enable you to select the best textbooks

Essential MCQs for Surgical Finals
Hassanally & Wasan
- The crucial material for your exam success
- Extended teaching notes, bullet points and mnemonics
- Revision indexes for easy access to specific topics

Essential MCQs for Medical Finals
Wasan, Hassanally & Wasan
- The crucial material for your exam success
- Extended teaching notes, bullet points and mnemonics
- Revision indexes for easy access to specific topics

For priority mail order service, please contact PasTest on 01565 752000, or ORDER ONLINE AT OUR SECURE WEBSITE.

PasTest Ltd, Egerton Court, Parkgate Estate, Knutsford, Cheshire WA16 8DX
Telephone: 01565 752000   Fax: 01565 650264
E-mail: books©pastest.co.uk Website: http//www.pastest.co.uk